1197

618·2

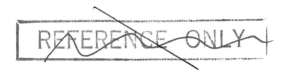
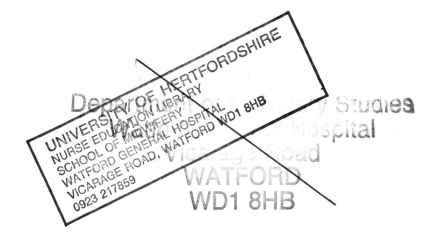

PREGNANCY CARE IN THE 1990s

PREGNANCY CARE
IN THE 1990s

Edited by Geoffrey Chamberlain and Luke Zander

The Proceedings of a Symposium held at

The Royal Society of Medicine

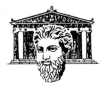

The Parthenon Publishing Group
International Publishers in Medicine, Science & Technology

Casterton Hall, Carnforth,
Lancs, LA6 2LA, UK

120 Mill Road, Park Ridge,
New Jersey 07656, USA

Published in the UK by
The Parthenon Publishing Group Limited
Casterton Hall, Carnforth,
Lancs, LA6 2LA, England

Published in the USA by
The Parthenon Publishing Group Inc.
120 Mill Road
Park Ridge,
New Jersey 07656, USA

British Library Cataloguing-in-Publication Data
Pregnancy Care in the 1990s: Proceedings of a Symposium
at the Royal Society of Medicine, April 1991
I.   Chamberlain, Geoffrey
II.   Zander, Luke
618.24

ISBN 1-85070-393-0

First published 1992

Lasertypesetting by Martin Lister Publishing Services, Bolton-le-Sands,
Carnforth, Lancs

Printed in Great Britain by The Cromwell Press Ltd, Melksham, Wiltshire

Contents

List of contributors   vii

Preface   ix

Foreword   xi

Section 1   Setting the scene

1   The changing social context of pregnancy care   3
    Ann Oakley

2   Appropriate pregnancy policies in the 1990s: an   19
    economic dimension
    Alan Maynard

3   Legal influences on clinical practice   31
    Robert Dingwall

4   The development of health care policies   41
    Chris Ham

    General discussion I   49

Section 2   Professional and public participation in policy-making

5   An obstetrician's view of the maternity services in the   59
    1990s
    Richard Beard

6   The midwife's contribution   67
    Margaret Brain

7   General practitioner participation in policy-making   75
    Peter Kielty

8   Priorities in maternity health care: a paediatric view   79
    Malcolm Levene

9   Participation in policy-making: the maternity service   83
    users
    Mary Newburn

10   A politician's views   93
     Renée Short

     General discussion II   97

**Section 3   To what extent have research findings influenced
     policies?**

11   Research findings and policy-making   113
     Barbara Stocking

12   The content and process of antenatal care   121
     Marion Hall

13   The basis of a midwifery team: continuity of carer   127
     Caroline Flint

14   Place of birth   137
     Gavin Young

15   Neonatal intensive care   147
     Richard Cooke

     General discussion III   153

Section 4   The way forward

16   Maternity services after 1992   161
     Rosemary Jenkins

17   Changing the training programme   169
     Wendy Savage

18   Making it happen: the politics of change   177
     Laurie McMahon

     General discussion IV   187

     Conclusions   197

     Index   199

List of contributors

Professor Richard Beard
Professor of Obstetrics
St Mary's Hospital
Praed Street
London   WC2 1NY

Miss Margaret Brain
President
Royal College of Midwives
15 Mansfield Street
London   W1M 0BE

Professor Geoffrey Chamberlain
Professor of Obstetrics &
   Gynaecology
St George's Hospital Medical School
Cranmer Terrace
London   SW17 0RE

Professor Richard Cooke
Professor of Child Health
Alder Hey Children's Hospital
Eaton Road
West Derby
Liverpool   L12 2AP

Professor Robert Dingwall
Professor of Social Studies
University of Nottingham Medical
   School
Queen's Medical Centre
Nottingham   NG7 2UH

Miss Caroline Flint
Independent Midwife
34 Elm Quay Court
Nine Elms Lane
Vauxhall
London   SW8 5DE

Miss Marion Hall
Consultant Obstetrician
Aberdeen Maternity Hospital
Cornhill Road
Aberdeen   AB9 2ZA

Professor Chris Ham
Fellow in Health Policy and
   Management
King's Fund College
2 Palace Court
London   W2 4HS

Miss Rosemary Jenkins
Professional Officer
RCM Welsh Board
Brandy Cove Suite
Microlink House
Queensway
Swansea Industrial Estate
Fforestfach
Swansea   SA5 4DJ

Dr Peter Kielty
General Practitioner
23 Leyton Road
Harpenden
Herts

Professor Malcolm Levene
Professor of Paediatrics & Child
   Health
Leeds General Infirmary
Great George Street
Leeds   LS1 3EX

Dr Laurie McMahon
Director of Organization Consultancy
Office of Public Management
Pyramid House
252B Grays Inn Road
London WC1X 8JR

Professor Alan Maynard
Director of the Centre for Health
 Economics
University of York
York

Miss Mary Newburn
Head of Policy and Development
National Childbirth Trust
Alexandra House
Oldham Terrace
London W3 6NH

Professor Ann Oakley
Social Science Research Unit
Institute of Education
University of London
55 Gordon Square
London WC1H 0NT

Sir George Pinker
President, Royal Society of Medicine
96 Harley Street
London W1N 1AF

Dr Wendy Savage
Senior Lecturer and Consultant
Department of Obstetrics
The London Hospital (Whitechapel)
Mile End
Bancroft Road
London E1

Mrs Renée Short
Past Chairman, Parliamentary Select
 Committee on Social Services
70 Westminster Gardens
Marsham Street
London SW1P 4JG

Miss Barbara Stocking
Director
King's Fund Centre
126 Albert Street
London NW1 7NF

Dr Gavin Young
Chairman
Association of Community based
 Maternity Care
Barn Croft
Temple Sowerby
Penrith
Cumbria CA10 1RZ

Dr Luke Zander
Senior Lecturer
Department of General Practice
United Medical and Dental Schools
 of Guys and St Thomas'
80 Kennington Road
London SE11

Preface

One of the disturbing characteristics of the contemporary medical scene is the steadily increasing fragmentation of the health care services, partly due to the inevitable increase in specialization. Contact and collaboration between individuals from different disciplines and specialty groups are becoming ever more difficult and the developing isolation within which many are now working has important and significant implications to both the planning and delivery of medical care.

In 1980 we convened a Conference at the Royal Society of Medicine entitled 'Pregnancy Care for the 1980s'. The meeting was unusual in that the participants were drawn from a wide range of differing disciplines including Obstetrics, General Practice, Midwifery, Paediatrics, the Behavioural Sciences, Education and also included representatives of the receivers of care. The success of the Conference was widely considered to have been largely due to the wide range of perspectives represented. The meeting served as a stimulus and catalyst for the subsequent establishment of the multidisciplinary Forum on Maternity and the Newborn, which is now firmly established at the Royal Society of Medicine.

When we were considering the content for its sequel 'Pregnancy Care in the 1990s', it would have been very natural to focus on topics which are at the forefront of the disciplines concerned with pregnancy care, and to consider the clinical and organizational developments that are likely to take place over the coming decade. However, we recognized that these are the issues which form the substance of many other meetings and conferences that we all attend in the course of our normal professional activities. We wanted this Conference to contribute something rather different to the deliberations in which all of us are engaged in our individual spheres of activity, as had been achieved by the previous one. Therefore, rather than choosing particular aspects of care, we thought it would be valuable to consider the more fundamental question of how to ensure that what we are doing is actually appropriate, a topic that is all too often neglected by those concerned with maternity care decision-making.

The best way to get full value from a multidisciplinary conference is to ensure that ample opportunity is provided for those with differing perspectives to share their views. A characteristic of this conference, as it is of all the Forum meetings, is that much time was given over to unstructured discussion and comment from the participants, as opposed to formal papers being followed by question and answer sessions. We have endeavoured to capture this sense of debate and interchange of views by including the essence of these discussions, together with the formal papers in this book of the proceedings. The success of the meeting clearly underlined the value of such communication and illustrated the benefits to be derived from such gatherings.

Acknowledgements

We should like to express our very sincere thanks to all the speakers who provided manuscripts so promptly and to our secretaries, Mrs Anne Fraser and Mrs Carmel Stephenson, for their work in producing the transcription. We would also like to thank Wyeth Laboratories for their financial support for the meeting.

Royal Society of Medicine *Luke Zander*
June 1992 *Geoffrey Chamberlain*

Foreword

This book records the proceedings of the second Conference held jointly at the Royal Society of Medicine, between the Section of Obstetrics and Gynaecology and the Forum on Maternity and the Newborn. The meeting clearly recaptured the enthusiasm generated in the first conference in 1980. The individual Forum papers are reported and the joint editors, both of whom are experienced authors and practising obstetricians of national repute, have distilled carefully the contents of a valuable debate following each group of papers.

The subjects chosen are central to the development of pregnancy care in the 1990s and none of the sensitive areas which are current between professionals responsible for this care were shirked; rather they were aired and debated freely. In the atmosphere of change which exists in the maternity services today, enquiry is recommended into the appropriateness of current educational programmes for maternity health care professionals.

This book emphasizes, in its choice of subjects and authors, the need for mutual respect between the various groups of maternity health care workers, respect for individual abilities, aspirations and the value of co-operative effort to ensure progress in change is properly emphasized. Due importance is given to the most basic and important factors in the equation, namely the mother's wishes and her professional needs.

The papers presented are from the nation's leaders in the various aspects of pregnancy care. The editors are to be congratulated on promoting this second look conference in a vital area of medicine and for the way in which they have contributed to and have responsibly drawn the threads together in this publication.

Royal Society of Medicine
March 1992

Sir George Pinker KCVO
President Elect

Section 1
Setting the scene

1

The changing social context of pregnancy care

Ann Oakley

In thinking about the future of maternity care, it is important to consider cultural values about childbirth, children, women, men and families; the social positions of mothers and fathers; the social positions of midwives and doctors; the social organization of maternity care; the role of health professionals and of the community in securing its own health; and the division of welfare between public and private sectors. This chapter focuses on three of these themes in particular:

(1) The demographic context within which maternity care is being, and will be, provided in the 1990s;

(2) The question of changes in family life;

(3) Issues concerning the ways in which those who use the maternity services are likely to interact with those who provide them: how will we build on the challenges and the struggles of the 1980s?

THE DEMOGRAPHIC CONTEXT

Projecting from the 1980s to the 1990s, a number of trends are clearly identifiable. To begin with, childbirth is becoming less popular. Between 1970 and 1987 in the UK the number of children per woman dropped from 2.44 to 1.82. In most other EC countries, the decrease was greater. Related to this, women's average age at first childbirth is rising: from 23.9 in 1970 to 26.4 years in 1987 for births within marriage, and from 24.5 in 1980 to 25.0 years in 1987 for all births. There are proportionately more births among older women. The proportion of women who never

3

have children is increasing; while 90% of those born in 1945 are mothers, this is expected to fall to 83% among women born in 1955. Again, similar trends are observable elsewhere in Europe. The birth rate is expected to peak in the early 1990s, when the large generation born in the 1960s is having children, and thereafter to decline[1].

These changes are occurring against a background of decreased provision of contraceptive services. The cuts in these services, and particularly the offloading of responsibility from family planning clinics to GPs, are serving to reduce women's choices. It is estimated that fewer than half of all GPs are trained to fit the cap or IUD[2] which, given the trend for oral contraception to become less popular[1], may pose something of a problem. Pregnancy terminations have been increasing since 1983. Between 1988 and 1989 there was a 14% rise. At the same time, regional differences in the availability of termination of pregnancy continue; in South Birmingham in 1988 only 1% of terminations carried out on women living in the district were within the NHS, whereas 99% of women in North Devon were able to get an NHS termination[2]. The increase in terminations is proportionately greater for younger women; here there has been a fourfold increase from the late 1960s to the late 1980s[3]. Indeed, the increased exposure of young women to the risks of pregnancy and childbirth is one of the most marked social trends of the 1980s. In the mid-1960s, 1 in 50 girls and 1 in 17 boys said they had had sexual intercourse before the age of 16. In 1988, these figures had risen to a striking 1 in 2 for girls and 1 in 3 for boys[4]. We can only speculate on the long-term impact of increasingly early sexual experience on conception, pregnancy and childbirth.

The second major change likely to continue into the 1990s is that the attractions of marriage as a context for childbirth appear to have worn thin. A total of 1 in 4 of all births are now to non-married women. This represents a fivefold increase in a decade[1], and is a new cultural pattern: before 1960 the proportion of births to non-married women had remained stable at about 4–5% for 50 years, with the exception of the two World Wars. In some areas today, for example inner London, more than 1 in 4 births now take place outside marriage, and the rate is substantially higher in some ethnic groups, particularly Afro-Caribbean women, where births outside marriage may soon exceed those within, making so-called legitimate babies the deviation rather than the norm. Indeed, this is already the case in Sweden. Within the EC, the UK has the fourth highest rate of births outside marriage. Our rate is also higher than that of the USA[1].

But it is not quite correct to say that marriage is no longer popular: in fact the UK also has the highest marriage rate in Europe. During the 1970s and 1980s the rate of marriage among men and women at ages 30 years and over remained more or less unchanged. It is among the young that the change has occurred, with only one-fifth the rate of marriages among the under-20s at the end of the 1980s compared to twenty years earlier[1]. As well as having the highest marriage rate, the UK also has the second highest divorce rate in Europe (Denmark is first).

OTHER CHANGES IN FAMILY LIFE

It is, of course, one thing to cite the statistics of birth and marriage, and quite another to interpret their meaning. On the surface at least, the declining popularity of marriage does not mean the disappearance of fathers. Along with the increase of births outside marriage has gone an increasing tendency for these to be registered by both parents. Whereas only 4% of live births outside marriage were registered by both parents in 1971, about 20% were so registered in 1989[1]. Many mothers who are not married to their children's fathers are living with those fathers. Nonetheless, these demographic and other changes have meant a decline in the traditional family – defined as a married couple living with their dependent children – as the context within which children are born and reared. Most people in the UK no longer live in such families. Over the last thirty years there has been a large increase both in single-person households, and in lone-parent families. The latter have more than doubled over this period. Of all families with dependent children, 1 in 7 is now a lone-parent family[1], and 1 in 5 children under 16 does not live with both his or her natural parents[2]. But in the midst of this change, there is also stability: 90% of all lone parents are women, a figure which has changed little over thirty years[2].

At the other end of the age range, long-term demographic changes resulting in an increase in the elderly as a group within the population also have an impact on family life, by increasing the amount of caring that has to be done within the community. The 1980 Women and Employment survey found that 1 in 8 adult women provided regular caring services for another adult, usually a parent or parent-in-law[5]. With the government policy of community care, which serves as a euphemism for women's unpaid caring services, this burden of dependency is likely to increase.

The mother of the 1990s is therefore more likely than her own mother to have children later and without being married, or, if married, to experience a change in her family circumstances precipitating her into lone motherhood. She is more likely to have other relatives to care for, as well as her own children. She is also considerably more likely to have paid employment of her own. Once again, the UK comes second to

Denmark in terms of having the highest economic activity rate for women. In more than half of all families with dependent children, both parents are employed[2]. A majority of mothers of dependent children are now employed, a figure which includes 40% of women with under-fives, rising to 75% of those whose youngest child is aged 11–15[1]. Structural changes in the distribution of jobs between different employment sectors mean that employment amongst women, including among mothers, is likely to rise further in the 1990s, becoming an important safety net to prevent families falling into poverty with the rise in male unemployment and the increase in lone motherhood. Some three-quarters of potentially poor households are moved out of poverty by women's earnings[6].

If this sounds as though mothers have too much to do, that is exactly the picture conveyed by division of labour and time budget surveys. In all households, women have less leisure time than men; for example, women in full-time employment enjoy 33 hours leisure per week compared with 44 hours for similarly employed men[1]. Other work has shown that the presence of a man in the household, irrespective of whether there are children or not, is what makes a difference to women's disposable time[7]. Time budget surveys show that 87% of the care provided for children under five is given by their mothers, and only 13% by their fathers[8]. The British Social Attitudes survey data on the division of labour between men and women in the home show almost no change over the 1980s in the gender distribution of household tasks[9]. For example, 5% of men made the evening meal in 1983 compared with 6% in 1987; 1% of men did the washing and the ironing in 1983 and 2% in 1987. A consistent finding of many studies is that men are more likely to say that they do more in the house than women say they do[9].

But whatever men's contribution to domestic labour, they are undoubtedly present in maternity care now in a way they were not thirty years ago, and there would seem to be no reason for this presence not to continue. From a more or less absolute ban at delivery in the late 1960s, we have now reached the point at which it is deviant for there not to be a man in the delivery room. Research carried out by Anne Woollett and colleagues[10] shows that before 1970 paternal attendance at birth was rare, but became the norm during that decade (see also Garcia and colleagues[11]). But whilst it is clear that men are expected to be in the delivery room, it remains unclear as to what they are supposed to do there[12,13].

Motherhood, and the ways in which mothers and babies are cared for or not, is not only a matter of fact, that is, of establishing what people do and how they do it. At the heart of many of our past, present and future dilemmas in this area is the conflict between expectations and ideals on the one hand, and reality on the other. This is a problem on a number of levels, including for women during the transition to mother-hood, who may find the contrast between the way they thought motherhood was going to be and the way it is quite literally depress-ing[14], and for children and young people exposed to school-based education for parenthood programmes, who are presented with a view of childbirth which by-passes the mother as main actor and is insensitive to emotional aspects of the experience[15]. But in these respects individual exposure merely mirrors cultural experience. More people hold to the notion of a proper family as one where the mother does not perform paid work than are willing (or able) to practise it. More people advocate the participation of fathers in family life and household work than live in egalitarian households. For example, in the British Social Attitudes survey caring for sick children equally was practised by 30% of married couples, but viewed prescriptively as an ideal by 51%[9].

Increasingly in the 1980s, and in the 1990s, the maternity services have had, and will have, to contend with the fact that Britain is an increasingly poor population, and the poorest groups in the population are women and children. Around 1 in 4 of all British children now live in or on the margins of poverty. Poverty is a fact of life for 7 out of 10 lone-parent families and for 2 out of 10 two-parent families. (Here poverty is defined as not above the old supplementary benefit or present income support level[8].) The reasons for this are complex. Important factors include the relative material disadvantage imposed on people through having children, the failure of marriage to protect women and children financially, and the culturally imposed inability of women as lone parents to provide for their children at the same level as is possible for men. For example, when one looks at the financial fates and likely futures of families with children compared to those without, the figures show a pattern of increasing inequality. Households with children are coming to occupy a proportionately larger share of the low-income band[16]. Between 1979 and 1985 in the bottom band of disposable income, the proportion of couples with children rose from 3 to 18%. Under the influence particularly of Thatcherite policies, the distribution of income and ownership of wealth have become increas-ingly unequal in the 1980s[1]. Increased male unemployment contributes, though in a quarter of poor families the family 'head' is in full-time work[1]. There has been a corresponding increase in homelessness: be-tween 1978 and 1989 there was a 240% increase in the number of homeless families in Britain[2].

Money is only one of a number of resources which contribute to health and well-being. Others, including space, time and food, also show a pattern of distribution which disadvantages women and children[17,18]. Some years ago the Maternity Alliance showed how the income of many families is unable to support an adequate diet for pregnant women, and this is likely to become increasingly the case in the future. Although pregnant women and young children need priority in the policy agenda, this is often not what happens, though the intention may not of course be to discriminate. For example, research on transport use shows the crucially declining availability of, but need for, low-cost public transport among women and children in low-income families.

Behind both the misfortunes of families, and the specific straits of female-headed lone-parent families, is the social position of women as mothers. Despite the efforts of feminism in the 1970s and 1980s, women's status in the public world remains secondary, and their role in the domestic world primary. Within the paid workforce they are far more likely to be in part-time, poorly paid, low status work than men; 80% of employed women are semi-skilled part-time workers[5]. Without social policy changes permitting a different domestic division of labour to emerge, women's unequal burden of caring work will remain and intensify during the 1990s. Using data from the 1980 Women and Employment survey, Heather Joshi has shown that a typical British mother who gives birth to and brings up two children will forego earnings of £122 000 over her lifetime. The lost earnings are consequent on a period of absence from the labour force, but part-time work and low paid work make a heavy contribution[7]. Since the lost earnings formula is sensitive to the interval between births – more earnings are foregone when the interval is larger – this fact may help to explain the tendency for intervals between births to decrease recently among UK mothers[1].

Women's work as childbearers and childrearers is performed mostly unpaid and in private, within the 'sanctity' of the home. A striking feature of British family life is the low level of provision for out-of-home childcare. Both in absolute and relative terms this is low, and the trend is towards less, not more. Less than 1% of British under-fives have access to local authority day nursery places, and less than 1% of primary school children are able to use out-of-school care facilities[2]. Although employer-provided crèches have received some media attention recently, a recent survey found only 198 out of 1.1 million women able to use these facilities[19]. In the European league the UK does badly, providing publicly funded childcare for only 2% of children under three, compared with 44% in Denmark, 25% in France, 5% in Italy and 4% in Portugal[2]. Since British children are as or more likely than their European counterparts to have no parent at home full-time to care for them, negotiating and resourcing childcare is a difficult business carried out on an individual basis and consisting of piecemeal packages of relatives, friends, neighbours and paid childminders for the majority of working parents, who cannot afford the middle-class convenience of a nanny[20].

THE FUTURE OF THE CONSUMER MOVEMENT

In their preface to *Pregnancy Care for the 1980s*, Luke Zander and Geoffrey Chamberlain observed that pregnancy care as a branch of medicine had recently become the focus of 'much debate and controversy in both medical and lay circles'[21]. Contentious issues had been raised in relation to objectives of care, the role of the consumer, and the contributions of the different professional groups. Subsequent chapters in the book addressed the following themes: the need to evaluate the effectiveness of antenatal care; consumer views; community-based initiatives; psychosocial aspects of childbirth and parent–child relationships; the advantages and disadvantages of home and hospital delivery; the roles of obstetrician, midwife and GP in modern obstetric care, and the desirability of preparation for parenthood programmes.

The period from the early 1970s to the late 1980s stands out as the era of the consumer movement in maternity care. There is no doubt that professionals providing maternity care have had to assimilate a sustained attack on their expertise. Beginning as a protest against high induction rates, this quickly generalized itself to become a complaint about the dominance of the medical model of childbirth, in which pregnancy is a pathology requiring institutionalization and care by high technology means, and women merely vessels for fetal transport – the best kind of incubator there is[22]. During these years a range of new maternity care pressure groups was set up, including the Maternity Alliance, the Stillbirth and Neonatal Death Society, the Foundation for the Study of Infant Deaths, the Pre-Eclamptic Toxaemia Society, and many others. Important new developments took place in the two older organizations, the Association for the Improvement of Maternity Services (AIMS) and the National Childbirth Trust (NCT). The voluntary organizations achieved some notable successes in focusing the attention of the public, professionals and policy-makers on specific questions in maternity care.

During a period when expenditure on health and social services is being curtailed, the role of pressure groups in helping the professionals to defend the resourcing of services is now critically important, as Lyn Durward and Ruth Evans[23] have pointed out. One important question is of course whether this is all merely lip service. What impact has the consumer movement had, and what is it likely to have in the 1990s? Here it would seem that the responsiveness of health professionals to the consumer demand for a more 'social' and participatory model of childbirth is at odds with several other important historical trends.

The first of these is the tendency within obstetrics, as the dominant profession dealing with childbirth, to assert the value of its own expert, interventionist perspective. Looking at the development of obstetrics over the whole period from the 1920s, Pamela Summey and Marsha Hurst[24,25] point out how the development of an interventionist ideology in the 1920s and 30s was linked with the need for obstetricians to differentiate themselves from general doctoring, and to establish links with the surgical specialty of gynaecology.

When the ideology of natural childbirth began to appear in the late 1940s, the challenge this at first posed to obstetrical expertise was met with a two-pronged strategy. Firstly, prepared women made better patients; a Presidential Address published in the *American Journal of Obstetrics* in 1955 even suggested that natural childbirth might succeed in replacing some of the confidence women had lost in their doctors[26]. Secondly, the profession began to take a decided interest in women's psyches, extending its professional domain by capturing a version of the psychosocial within it, and putting forward various new versions of old arguments, including the idea that women who 'failed' at reproduction had a deep-seated desire to be men, and that dissatisfaction with maternity care was a manifestation of an underlying rejection of womanhood, which in turn was one of the many malignant products of women's higher education.

When the new consumer movement arrived in the 1970s, a different set of responses was in evidence. Control and management came to be emphasized less than monitoring and surveillance. More significantly, however, women began to lose their central role as obstetrical patients, and the professional gaze shifted to the fetus.

It is increasingly argued in medicolegal circles, both in the USA and in Europe, that pregnant women cannot be considered to be the guardians of their unborn children's best interests. In the USA, women are being sued for behaviour during pregnancy believed to damage the unborn, and for refusing to consent to obstetrical procedures deemed by obstetricians to be required in the interests of the unborn's health. The development of the fetal rights movement threatens any partnership of childbearing women and health professionals that has been achieved, by proposing that women are not important in securing a good outcome of pregnancy. As the sociologist Barbara Katz Rothman[27] has argued, fetal rights go hand in hand with a growing tendency for 'commodification' in maternity care, which includes genetic counselling, and the screening and testing of fetuses as a form of 'quality control'. In this process, pregnant women are redefined as unskilled workers on a reproductive assembly line, and the tendency is to blame them for 'defective' products. Thus, most health education in pregnancy is individualistic, and based on the assumption that health-damaging lifestyles can easily be changed, rather than taking account of the evidence about the health-damaging effects of poverty, domestic violence and other social factors.

The commodification process is seen very clearly in the treatment of infertility, where modern techniques allow for the removal and insertion of body parts, and for the mixing of different bodies, in a way which would have been viewed as pure science fiction fifty or even twenty years ago. Though the development and application of these newer reproductive technologies proceeds outside the main field of maternity care, it is important to consider the needs of the involuntarily childless as well as those who do not have to tangle with the awful dilemmas of *in vitro* fertilization (IVF) and its like. It seems unlikely that the 1990s will see any increase in work on the primary prevention of infertility, that much noted missing agenda item.

Furthermore, the increasing use of IVF and related technologies inserts the technological imperative back into the heart of maternity care. Other incentives are relevant here, including the rise in private obstetric care with its associated higher intervention rate. Hospital In-Patient Enquiry data for 1985 showed that 10% of women delivering under the NHS, 17% delivering in amenity beds, and 23% of those using pay beds had Caesarean sections[28]. Legal influences on clinical practice are considered later in this volume, but are undoubtedly highly significant as forces pulling the profession away from any sensitivity, developed during the 1970s and 1980s, to the desire of many women to avoid intervention. The trebling of claims since late 1989 for compensation following birth injuries, hailed by a leading firm of health authority lawyers[29], draws attention to the importance of introducing a no-fault compensation scheme.

One of the criticisms made by consumers in the 1970s was of the kind of communication that characterizes maternity care encounters. It was said with good evidence[30,31], that the typical encounter between pregnant women and obstetricians and midwives prevented many women from voicing their questions and anxieties. The spectre of the Guardian-reading middle-class woman as the sole possessor of information-seeking qualities was laid to rest by Ann Cartwright's survey of induction in 1979[32], which showed the only class difference to reside in the articulation of questions: working-class women had more unasked, and therefore unanswered, questions than their middle-class peers. The extent to which maternity care encounters retain their traditional hierarchical format is not known, though the same themes have been thrown up repeatedly in surveys over the years. One of the developments that has not happened as a result of the consumer critique is regular monitoring of women's satisfaction with the maternity services[33]. In the British Social Attitudes survey, which includes a question about general satisfaction with the NHS, the 1988 report showed a substantial decrease in satisfaction since 1983: among women aged 18–34, there was a 17% rise in dissatisfaction, with 40% in 1987 saying they were very or quite dissatisfied with the NHS[9].

Systematic research on user satisfaction is, therefore, one aspect of maternity care that requires attention in the 1990s. Another is medical education, and the perspectives that doctors bring to the care they provide for childbearing women. Although it may be widely believed that some of the rampant sexism of earlier decades is now missing, the evidence does not support this[34]. Both in the USA and the UK, a major unmet challenge before the maternity services is to provide a type of care which does not reinforce gender, class and race inequalities. To do this will require more than the education of health professionals out of the repetition of outmoded stereotypes. Ann Phoenix and others have pointed out how some basic maternity care practices are racially discriminatory in their effects; for example, all newborn babies in the UK are routinely screened for phenylketonuria, which has an incidence of about 1 in 10 000 births, but is considerably more common in white than black populations, whereas newborn babies are not screened for conditions such as sickle cell disease which affect mostly black populations; an estimated 1 in 200 babies of Caribbean origin and 1 in 100 of those of West African origin are born with sickle cell disease[35].

CONCLUSION

In summary, pregnancy care in the 1990s will need to contend with a social context in which childbearing women and their families are themselves having to struggle against considerable social and economic odds. More pregnant women and more children will in future be economically dependent on themselves and on the state. The consequences of the health and social policies of the last ten years amount to a dismantling of the welfare state, which was set up in part to protect the health of this vulnerable group. Unless it is restored, however caring is the antenatal work of midwives, GPs and obstetricians, they will increasingly have to function without the safety net of other support services.

Secondly, those who provide maternity care will need to bear in mind the decreasing likelihood that the pregnant women they care for live in traditional families. The notion that behind every pregnant woman there is a supportive husband lurking and ready to supply emotional companionship, domestic help and financial resources, will increasingly be a piece of cultural mythology. The old label 'marital status' is becoming a poorer guide to women's living circumstances. Whether a woman is legally married or not does not inform her health care providers, either about her household arrangements, or as to the social and financial support available to her. Within the context of a multicultural society, it is especially important that health care providers do not make any implicit or explicit judgements about conventional family arrangements. Similarly, it is important to be aware that there is no evidence that non-traditional family arrangements are health-damaging contexts for children. The poorer health outcomes observed in lone-parent and young mother households, for example, are a consequence of poverty, and not of some adverse effect that follows from membership of such families.

Thirdly, whilst the consumer movement will not go away, neither will other important influences on the shape of maternity care. We live in a world which values technology, and which has relinquished control over many aspects of life to professionals. The pressure on obstetricians to maintain an interventionist pose, and to maintain complex, perhaps unevaluated monitoring and surveillance systems, is likely to be intense. In view of this, the role of midwives and GPs in defending normality in pregnancy will be crucial. So, too, will be the systematic evaluation of the effectiveness, appropriateness and safety of different treatments and procedures within maternity care, which is, along with the consumer movement, the greatest heritage of the 1970s.

Finally, in the future development of maternity care it will be essential to bear in mind the single most important message of the consumer movement: that pregnancy is above all a social relationship. This relationship, rather than its fragmentation into parts owned by different experts or fought over by the courts, or jeopardized by poverty and material deprivation, remains the main challenge for the development of appropriate care in the 1990s: how to respect the integrity and autonomy of each woman and baby in their own, unique social context, while at the same time using the best endeavours and most appropriate resources of the health care system to provide safe, sensitive and effective care.

REFERENCES

1. Central Statistical Office. (1991). *Social Trends 21*. (London: HMSO)
2. Coote, A., Harman, H. and Hewitt, P. (1990). *The Family Way, Social Policy Paper No 1*. (London: Institute for Public Policy Research)
3. 1990. One in five pregnancies aborted as terminations reach record. *The Guardian*, 20th Sept
4. Estaugh, V. and Wheatley, J. (1990). *Family Planning and Family Well-being, Occasional Paper No 12*. (London: Family Policy Studies Centre)
5. Martin, J. and Roberts, C. (1984). *Women and Employment: A Lifetime Perspective*. (London: HMSO)
6. Morris, L. (1990). *The Workings of the Household*, p. 137. (Cambridge: Polity Press)
7. Joshi, H. (1987). *The Cash Opportunity Costs of Childbearing: an Approach to Estimation using British Data, Discussion Paper No. 208*. (London: Centre of Economic Policy Research)
8. Kiernan, K. and Wicks, M. (1990). *Family Change and Future Policy*, p. 30. (London: Family Policy Studies Centre)
9. Jowell, R., Witherspoon, S. and Brook, L.(eds.) (1988). *British Social Attitudes: the 5th Report*. (London: Gower)
10. Woollett, A., White, D. and Lyon, L. (1982). Observations of fathers at birth. In Beail, N. and McGuire, J. (eds.) *Fathers: Psychological Perspectives*. (London: Junction Books)
11. Garcia, J., Corry, M., MacDonald, D., Albourne, D. and Grant, A. (1985). Mothers' views of continuous electronic fetal heart monitoring and intermittent auscultation in a randomized controlled trial. *Birth*, 12, 79–85
12. Barbour, R.S. (1990). Fathers: the emergence of a new consumer group. In Garcia, J., Kilpatrick, R. and Richards, M. (eds.) *The Politics of Maternity Care*, pp. 202–16. (Oxford: Oxford University Press)
13. Richman, J., Goldthorp, W.O. and Simmons, C. (1975). Fathers in Labour. *New Society*, 16 October
14. Oakley, A. (1980). *Women Confined: Towards a Sociology of Childbirth*. (Oxford: Martin Robertson)
15. Prendergast, P. and Prout, A. (1990). Learning about birth: parenthood and sex education in English secondary schools. In Garcia, J. In Garcia, J., Kilpatrick, R. and Richards, M. (eds.) *The Politics of Maternity Care*, pp. 133–48. (Oxford: Oxford University Press)
16. Roll, J. (1988). *Family Fortunes: Parents' Incomes in the 1980s, Occasional Paper No. 7*. (London: Family Policy Studies Centre)
17. Pahl, J. (1989). *Money and Marriage*. (London: Macmillan)
18. Charles, N. and Kerr, M. (1988). *Women, Food and Families*. (Manchester: University Press)
19. *The Independent*. Firms failing to provide childcare. 9.4.90
20. Brannen, J. and Moss, P. (1990). *Managing Mothers*. (London: Unwin Hyman)
21. Zander, L. and Chamberlain, G. (eds.) (1984). Preface. *Pregnancy Care for the 1980s*. (London: Macmillan)

14

22. Oakley, A. (1984). *The Captured Womb: a History of Antenatal Care in Britain.* (Oxford: Blackwells)
23. Durward, L. and Evans, R. (1990). Pressure groups and maternity care. In Garcia, J., Kilpatrick, R. and Richards, M. (eds.) *The Politics of Maternity Care,* pp. 256–73. (Oxford: Oxford University Press)
24. Summey, P.S. and Hurst, M. (1986). Ob/Gyn on the rise: the evolution of professional ideology in the twentieth century – Part 1. *Women and Health,* **11 (1),** 133–45
25. Summey, P.S. and Hurst, M. (1986). Ob/Gyn on the rise: the evolution of professional ideology in the twentieth century – Part 2. *Women and Health,* **11 (2),** 103–22
26. Mack, H.C. (1955). Back to Sacajawea. Presidential Address. *Am. J. Obstet. Gynecol.,* **69,** 933–49
27. Rothman, B.K. (1989). *Recreating Motherhood: Ideology and Technology in Patriarchal Society.* (New York: W.W. Norton)
28. Macfarlane, A. (1988). Holding back the tide of caesareans (letter). *Br. Med. J.,* **297,** 852
29. 1990. NHS faces crisis over birth claims. *The Guardian,* 18th Oct
30. Fisher, S. (1986). *In the Patient's Best Interests: Woman and the Politics of Medical Decisions.* (New Jersey: Rutgers University Press)
31. Roberts, H. (1985). *Patient Patients: Women and Their Doctors.* (London: Pandora Press)
32. Cartwright, A. (1979). *The Dignity of Labour?* (London: Tavistock)
33. Jacoby, A. and Cartwright, A. (1990). Finding out about the views and experiences of maternity-service users. In Garcia, J., Kilpatrick, R. and Richards, M. (eds.) *The Politics of Maternity Care,* pp. 238–55. (Oxford: Oxford University Press)
34. Hawkins, J.W. and Aber, C.S. (1988). The content of advertisements in medical journals: distorting the image of women. *Women and Health,* **14 (2),** 43–59
35. Phoenix, A. (1990). Black women and the maternity services. In Garcia, J., Kilpatrick, R. and Richards, M. (eds.) *The Politics of Maternity Care,* pp. 274–99. (Oxford: Oxford University Press)

DISCUSSION

Bill Lindsay (Upjohn Ltd.)   I was very interested in the break-up of the family and the 90% rate of women who now look after children; society almost dictates that this is so and it would be a very brave woman who actually leaves her children. This may be the reason why there are not many husbands looking after their children.

Christine Gowdridge (Maternity Alliance)   We would not laugh at statistics on poverty of women, or those that show 1 in 4 babies is born poor, but we do laugh at the statistics showing that 1% of men do the ironing, that 13% of men care for their children and there is a clear link between these two statistics. If only 1% of men are doing the ironing, it is not because they are out on the street campaigning for maternity leave.

Iain Chalmers (National Perinatal Epidemiology Unit, Oxford)   There may have been a mistake in the example quoted from Ann Phoenix. The incidence of phenylketonuria is 1 in 10 000. It clearly differs from sickle trait for there is a clear intervention, that is avoidance of food with phenylalanine, which should be adopted in those cases shown to be positive.

Wendy Savage (Obstetrician, London)   In that example, thalassaemia occurs in Europeans who are not from the Mediterranean in about 1 in 500, so it would seem logical to screen for that and yet we do not and I think that is a point that did not come over.

Professor Malcolm Levene (Paediatrician, Leeds)   The point about screening is that it is only valuable if you also have treatment that can be used prior to the patient exhibiting symptoms; for phenylalanine, he develops convulsions and mental retardation. In the other examples that are cited (for example, sickle cell disease, thalassaemia and cystic fibrosis) these conditions can be screened for, but there is not the same possibility to intervene early and then prevent the disease. This is the most important thing, not racial groups or biological higher risk but that adequate and appropriate intervention to prevent the disease is available. The decision of parents must also be borne in mind. There are some parents who regard screening as important, even if there is no simple obvious intervention.

Mary Newburn (National Childbirth Trust)   I was very interested in the third theme that you talked about: the user/provider relationship. You referred to £30 million funding for user organizations; this includes the voluntary organizations, not just the maternity care groups. The core funding the NCT is getting this year from the Department of Health is £12 000; halfway through the 1980s it was £30 000; it is actually going down.

Rona Scandall (Director, Stillbirth and Neonatal Death Society)   Our Government money has decreased from 57 to 11% of core funding this year. I do not feel confident about the role of voluntary organizations in consumer groups, for such a lot of our time is spent fighting for money. We hope that consumers of maternity services realize that it is not only successful outcomes of pregnancies that are important to women. It is also what happens when they miscarry or when their babies are born dead.

Doris Shaw (Midwife, New York)   The Assistant Secretary of Health of the USA recently announced that one of the best infant outcomes in the United States was among Mexican-American women. These are ladies who usually do not take advantage of prenatal care until late in pregnancy; they do tend to be married, to be older when they become pregnant and tend not to smoke; it shows that the lifestyle of the woman has a lot to do with the infant.

Luke Zander (General Practitioner, London)   It is not so much a question of what should we do but how should we do it? Working in primary care and in midwifery in the community is a topic that we need to look at very carefully. If the people for whom we are providing care are going to have so many social disadvantages, this issue is terribly important.

Professor Ann Oakley   I did not mean to be depressing, though I am often accused of that. I meant to draw attention to some of the things that are happening in this country, of which many maternity care providers are not sufficiently aware. For example, pregnant women are often told to go home and rest. It always seems to me that piece of advice does not take account of the conditions of pregnant women's lives; there is good evidence that women, when told to go home and rest, actually work harder than those who are not given that advice. I was trying to introduce a note of reality about the kinds of lives that pregnant women actually lead.

Ann Rider (Maternity Services Manager, London)   How do we actually get these ideas into practice? With the new NHS arrangements, the Health Authority becomes the purchaser who can demand the type of service that is required; here is the authority that we should be lobbying and informing about getting maternity care into woman's social context, giving her greater autonomy. We have made some strides towards continuity of care and that is what we have to keep doing. Without continuity of care, how can you actually elicit the woman's real needs and her social support, and encourage her to take autonomy for her care. As a Director of Midwifery, I am worried about our service. Have midwives got the communication skills to sustain good continuity care? I leave others to comment on the communication skills of the medical staff.

Rosemary Jenkins (Midwife, Royal College of Midwives)   Your presentation and the discussion have looked at the way we should be altering our care, but if poverty is one of the main determinants of the outcome of maternity care, should we not perhaps be looking outwardly at the political stances the professionals should also make? Two specific areas relating to this are:

(1)   The offer from Europe of a social charter that goes some way towards making statements about levels of income, which to date has been almost entirely rejected by our Government.

(2)   There is a draft EEC directive on pregnant women and the benefits that should be available to them under EEC law. That is far more advantageous than what is available to women today in this country. Should we not be moving to adopt outside pressure in order to get at poverty?

2

Appropriate pregnancy policies in the 1990s: an economic dimension

Alan Maynard

INTRODUCTION

Health care is only one of many factors which influence the health of infants and mothers. Indeed it is likely that for many at-risk infants and mothers the redistribution of income, involving increased support from social security programmes, would enhance their health more at a given cost than investing further resources in the NHS. Whilst it is essential to bear this fact in mind, the focus of this chapter is to address the issue of prioritization in the health service: which treatments for which episodes generate the greatest increase in the health of recipients at least cost, and how will the increased production of these data affect decision-making in the NHS in the 1990s?

WHY WE HAVE TO SET PRIORITIES

The basis of economics is that demand is infinite and the supply of resources is finite. As a consequence decision-makers, be they individuals, families, institutions or nations, have to decide how to allocate limited resources among many competing activities. Any choice to invest scarce resources involves an opportunity cost: a decision to treat one infant means that resources are consumed which could have been used to treat another patient. There are insufficient resources to treat all patients and, as a consequence, some mothers and infants will be denied treatments from which they could benefit.

As a consequence of the need to allocate resources carefully, sometimes referred to as rationing, it is essential to identify those treatments which give the greatest health benefit, measured in terms of enhancements in the length and quality of life of the mother or infant who is treated, at least cost. Because resources are limited and all choices involve opportunity costs, it is necessary to target resources on those activities which produce 'the biggest bang for the buck'.

HOW TO SET PRIORITIES

What criteria should be used to decide which patients will be treated and which mothers and infants will not be treated? The alternatives are allocation on the basis of willingness and ability to pay and allocation on the basis of 'need'. Even Mrs Thatcher rejected the idea that access to health care should be determined by ability to pay, saying:

'the principle that adequate health care should be provided for all, regardless of their ability to pay, must be the foundation of any arrangement for financing health care'.

The alternative, access to care on the basis of patient need, is ambiguous unless a clear definition of need is agreed. If need is defined as the patients' ability to benefit, measured in terms of improved health per unit of cost, the effective functioning of such a system of health care requires good information about the cost and health benefits of alternative treatments so that managers, both clinical and non-clinical, can demonstrate that they use resources efficiently and meet patients' needs.

IMPROVING INFORMATION AND THE REFORMED NHS

All healthcare systems, including the NHS, are run in the absence of relevant data about inputs (costs), activities (processes of treatment and care), and outcomes (improvements in patient health). Indeed, the Government's 'redisorganization' of the NHS has, if anything, worsened the supply of information due to the failures of the Korner information system and the inefficient investment in information technology which has accompanied the 1990–91 reform of the NHS.

The data that are available suggest that there are significant variations in practice and outcomes. The cost data available now, and the pricing data that will be available in 1991 and beyond are poor measures of opportunity costs. Decisions about how to treat and who to treat are made in 'a data-free environment' and on the basis of guesses rather than sound knowledge of the costs and outcomes of competing treatments.

There is not only an ignorance about cost–outcome relationships, with most therapies in use in the NHS unproven, there is also an absence of appropriate incentives to induce decisions to seek and use the results of economic evaluation. The Government is seeking to mitigate this problem by separating out the demand (purchaser) and supply (provider) sides of the market and requiring these 'actors' to contract for services. The purchaser is required to prioritize treatments on the basis of cost-effectiveness and if providers do not seek and use such data to improve their practices, they may fail to win purchaser contracts and, in the limit, go out of business.

If successful, the reformed NHS will lead to more data being produced about the cost-effectiveness of competing treatments. The contracting process may induce decision-makers to use such information and improve the efficiency with which resources are used.

GLASNOST AND PERESTROIKA: WILL THEY WORK?

Greater openness in contracting and the restricting of incentives may enhance efficiency. Glasnost will make explicit the rationing of care, which is now ubiquitous but implicit. This transparency in decision-making should enhance accountability. However, a brief review of history indicates we have been here before, that is, the need to measure outcomes and manage resources systematically has been noted for many centuries, and ignored. Francis Clifton, physician to the Prince of Wales, in 1732, argued:

'In order, therefore to procure this valuable collection, I humbly propose, first of all, that three or four persons should be employed in the hospitals (and that without any ways interfering with the gentlemen now concerned), to set down the cases of the patients there from day to day, candidly and judiciously, without any regard to private opinions or public systems, and at the year's end publish these facts just as they are, leaving every one to make the best use he can for himself'[1].

The editor of *The Lancet* in 1841–2 argued:

'All public institutions must be compelled to keep case-books and registers, on an uniform plan. Annual abstracts of the results must be published. The annual medical report of cases must embrace hospitals, lying-in hospitals, dispensaries, lunatic asylums, and prisons'[2].

His advice facilitated the passing of the Lunacy Act 1844 which required the managers of all public psychiatric hospitals to evaluate patient care in terms of whether the recipient was dead, relieved or unrelieved.

Florence Nightingale advocated the use of these categories in all hospitals and continued:

> 'I am fain to sum up with an urgent appeal for adopting this or some uniform system of publishing the statistical records of hospitals. There is a growing conviction that in all hospitals, even in those which are best conducted, there is a great and unnecessary waste of life. In attempting to arrive at the truth, I have applied everywhere for information, but in scarcely an instance have I been able to obtain hospital records fit for any purpose of comparison. If they could be obtained, they would enable us to decide many other questions besides the ones alluded to. They would show subscribers how their money was being spent, what amount of good was really being done with it, or whether the money was doing mischief rather than good'[3].

Data about dead, relieved or unrelieved patients were collected in many UK hospitals in the 19th century but these practices no longer exist and the ethos of outcome measurement is being recreated.

Will this regeneration of outcome measurement and the recognition of its central importance in managing pregnancy and other policies in the 1990s survive? There are reasons to believe that the use of cost–outcome measures to prioritize treatments is unavoidable throughout the world and that the formulation of pregnancy policies in the 1990s will be confused by facts!

PRIORITIES IN TREATMENTS: SOME PRELIMINARY ATTEMPTS

How much should be spent on what pregnancy services for which patients in the 1990s? The economic approach to answering this question is to identify those treatments which give the greatest health benefits (for example, years of life of good quality or quality-adjusted life years (QALYs) at least cost).

The following data are needed to identify low cost per QALY treatments:

(1)   Cost per treatment episode;

(2)   Length of survival;

(3)   Quality of survival (that is, ways of describing the quality of life measured in terms such as physical, social and psychological functioning);

(4)   Valuations of different combinations of descriptions of physical, social and psychological functioning; and

(5)   Agreement about the weighting of additional years of life or QALYs, at different times of the life cycle. (Is an additional year of life for an infant or mother more valuable to society than a year of life to an 85-year-old man or woman?)

All outcome and cost data are defective. The health and social care system is fragmented: primary care, hospital care, local authority social services and household social care operate within separate budgets and linking data to cost a treatment episode is difficult. Survival (mortality) data are also fragmented and poor. There is no gold standard quality of life measure and much disagreement about the merits and weaknesses of competing instruments. Despite these difficulties, crude guesstimates of the costs of producing one year of good quality life (a QALY) indicate that hip replacements produce a QALY at a cost less than that of producing the same benefit from dialysis for patients with chronic renal failure (see Table 1).

In the state of Oregon in the USA, the use of expert opinions, social preferences elicited from participants in public meetings and from a telephone survey, together with the judgements of the members of a State Health Care Commission have produced a priority listing of 714 procedures for the Medicaid programme[10]. Some items in this priority list are set out in Table 2. This shows that with decreasing birth weight the less likely it is that treatments will be funded.

The scientific base of the Oregon listing is weak but it is a powerful political statement of an intent to allocate resources explicitly and relate the funding of competing treatments to their social value.

The consequences of this approach in the USA and the UK will be profound. There will be a stronger incentive to evaluate practices more often and more rigorously. There will be a stronger incentive to use the results of such work to prioritize treatments: the managers will have an explicit rationale for their choices.

Table 1 The cost per quality-adjusted life year (QALY) of competing therapies: some tentative estimates from different sources*

Therapy	Cost/QALY (£, August 1990)
Cholesterol testing and diet therapy only (all adults, aged 40–69)	200[4]
Neurosurgical intervention for head injury	240[5]
GP advice to stop smoking	270[6]
Neurosurgical intervention for subarachnoid haemorrhage	490[7]
Antihypertensive therapy to prevent stroke (ages 45–64)	940[6]
Pacemaker implantation	1 100[7]
Hip replacement	1 180[7]
Valve replacement for aortic stenosis	1 410[7]
Cholesterol testing and treatment (all adults, aged 40–69)	1 480[4]
Coronary artery bypass grafting (left main vessel disease, severe angina)	2 090[7]
Kidney transplant	4 710[7]
Breast cancer screening	5 780[8]
Heart transplantation	7 840[7]
Cholesterol testing and treatment (incrementally) of all adults aged 25–39	14 150[4]
Home haemodialysis	21 970[7]
Coronary artery bypass grafting (vessel disease, moderate angina)	18 830[7]
Hospital haemodialysis	17 260[7]
Erythropoietin treatment for anaemia in dialysis patients (assuming a 10% reduction in mortality)	54 380[9]
Neurosurgical intervention for malignant intracranial tumours	107 780[5]
Erythropoietin treatment for anaemia in dialysis patients (assuming no increase in survival)	126 290[9]

* Superscript numbers indicate reference used as source

Table 2 Some examples of the Oregon priorities

Condition	Position on priority list
Pneumococcal pneumonia	1
Tuberculosis	2
Peritonitis	3
Low birth weight (1250 g and over)	23
Low birth weight (1000–1249 g)	73
Low birth weight (500–749 g)	358
Liver cirrhosis	695
Terminal HIV, with 10% chance of 5-year survival	707
Low birth weight (less than 500 g, under 23 weeks gestation)	713

CONCLUSIONS

The 1991 redisorganization of the NHS has created, in the separation of the provider and purchaser functions, a structure in which in principle at least, the criteria for allocating resources will be explicit and related to guesstimates of costs and outcome. There are some pregnancy services of unproven and dubious value. In the 1990s purchasers may cease to fund these services, shifting resources to those which are more defensible in terms of the costs of producing health improvements (QALYs). Explicit decisions not to treat, for instance, especially low birth weight infants will raise social, ethical and political as well as economic issues. The scarcity of resources makes such rationing inevitable. In the 1990s the rationing process will become more explicit and controversial as purchasers decide which mothers and infants will be deprived of care and who will be treated.

REFERENCES

1. Clifton, F. (1732). *The State of Physick Ancient and Modern, Briefly Considered.* (London)
2. Editorial (1840–41). *Lancet*, 650–1
3. Nightingale, F. (1863). *Some Notes on Hospitals.* (London: Longmans)
4. Department of Health Standing Medical Advisory Committee. (1990). *Blood Cholesterol Testing: the Cost-effectiveness of Opportunistic Cholesterol Testing.*
5. Pickard, J.D., Bailey, S., Sanderson, H., Rees, M. and Garfield, J.S. (1990). Step towards cost–benefit analysis of regional neurosurgical care. *Br. Med. J.*, 301, 629–35

6. Teeling Smith, G. (1990). The economics of hypertension and stroke. *Am. Heart J.*, **119**, 3, Part 2 (Suppl.), 725–8
7. Williams, A. (1985). Economics of coronary artery bypass grafting. *Br. Med. J.*, **249**, 326–9
8. Department of Health and Social Security, Forrest Report. (1986). *Breast Cancer Screening*. (London: HMSO)
9. Hutton, J., Leese, B. and Maynard, A. (1990). The Cost-effectiveness of the Use of Erythropoietin in the Treatment of Anaemia Arising from Chronic Renal Failure. *Occasional Paper*, University of York
10. Health Services Commission (1991). *Prioritized Health Services List*, February 20, 1991, Salem, Oregon

DISCUSSION

Deborah Kroll (Midwife Teacher, London) One of the difficulties with discussion and argument about economy and efficiency in the maternity care service is the way we currently provide it. How do you begin to cost and evaluate a service when there is duplication and even triplication of care by GP, midwives and obstetricians, with a persistent under-utilization of care by midwives, the ideal providers of care for healthy pregnant women?

Professor Alan Maynard (Director, Centre for Health Economics, York) I am involved in a Health Authority in the North and recognize the problems that you are putting forward. In making choices about how you put money into particular areas, it is important to have better knowledge about the impact of those particular services on patients' health. It is possible to design trials which look at different ways of treating and looking after patients; then we would have better information and might be able to make informed choices.

Adam Foreman (General Practitioner, Sheffield) Although they are crude, the evaluation and measurement of the maternity services have always been there. What has been going on in health economics in the 1980s has continued to make a commodity of childbearing, trying to squeeze the whole issue of health care into some kind of cost–benefit analysis.

The data about which we should be worried relate to how poverty affects health. There were quite clear figures in the Black Report on 'The Inequalities of Health'. Much of the attempt to try to make health care a commodity is a smoke-screen to cover those things which are basically getting worse and worse. We should be trying to address making health care a society issue and not an individual one; you have been describing the individualizing of health care problems.

Professor Maynard It depends on what question you ask. If the question is, how to allocate resources in the NHS between different areas, the sort of approach that I have been talking about is appropriate. We have to look at where you get the best benefit to patients when spending your money. If the question is, what is the best way of improving the health of mothers and children, then you are right that it would probably be a good idea to sack a few GPs and midwives and spend the money on social security.

Jilly Rosser (Institute of Child Health, Bristol) If one were able to get the necessary information, could we find out how £1000 was best spent in preventing, for example, preterm birth? The system described may at best enable us to choose between a day of neonatal intensive care or screening all pregnant women for infections at 24 weeks and giving them antibiotics or social interventions of the type that Ann Oakley has described, which may be able to increase the birth weight by 125 grams at best. The system still does not enable us to consider any of the other things that Ann Oakley talked about. If £1000 is better spent on the pregnant woman having a better diet or living in bed and breakfast accommodation, it does not seem that we have moved any closer towards improving that situation.

Professor Maynard   I think it depends on what you mean by improvement in the situation. If we can actually identify a particular programme of social security which enhances the woman's access to funds and we can observe certain health outcomes for her and her children, then we have moved quite a considerable way. I think the basic problem is that we still argue about these things on the basis of value. We could, in principle, evaluate whether to put money into prevention or into treatment.

Miranda Mugford (Health Economist, Oxford)   The main thing that health economists note is the problem of information. Within the field of maternity care, we are very fortunate for we have the Oxford Database of Perinatal Trials. It is not comprehensive, for everything has not been evaluated, but it is far advanced compared to other aspects of health care and includes evaluation of practices which are not just health care practices. We were looking forward to the new Korner information systems that, it was promised, were going to gather together national data about the maternity services. These have not materialized and now 1985 is the most recent year for which there are data about maternity care in maternity hospitals in England and Wales. It does not look as though it is going to get better very soon.

Marion Hall (Obstetrician, Aberdeen)   You emphasized that you were only talking about episodes of care. Some health problems do occur conveniently in episodes, such as much of general surgery; the system applies to some extent to pregnancy, for it is a self-limiting condition but there are much longer-lasting implications, some lasting a lifetime. For example, the birth of a child with Down's Syndrome carries with it all sorts of consequences in the future, and having a Caesarean section in one birth has implications for the next pregnancy. Health care cannot be so conveniently divided into episodes, but the present arrangements for spending money on health are short-termist. With the devolution of budgets, people are concerned with short-term efficiency; what is being called efficiency is actually often moving something onto somebody else's budget. I doubt whether the pricing mechanisms or the costing mechanisms are adequate to allow the people who are purchasing health care to make the appropriate choices.

Professor Maynard Short-termism is a real problem and always has been. In any health care system where people can push patients onto other people's budgets. There are often very sharp incentives to do that if you have got a cash-limited budget. The present arrangements actually accentuate the cost-shifting.

You are right about episodes; it is very difficult to define what an episode is. What I was trying to do was to emphasize that in looking at any studies you must be very careful about what period of time is being analysed because it may affect the results quite significantly.

Tony Golding (Public Health Doctor, London) I am sure what you have described is the right way forward, to analyse and divide each cost, but I am alarmed at the implications. If you take the Oregon figures which mean that public money should not be spent on babies under 750 grams, is the implication that private monies can be? Will you gradually get a two-tier system whereby the public hospitals in this country, if they adopt that system, can provide the same sort of care that is given privately? This would be a major change and it seems to me an implication, not only about babies but to the whole quality approach.

Professor Maynard The implication of both Oregon and of any other approach to rationing is that you make explicit who you are not going to treat. It would identify particularly vulnerable groups who would be deprived of care. That is exactly what is being done in our system but in a variety of covert ways. What it has lead to is a leakage of patients across jurisdictions, so patients in Oregon are trying to get their liver transplants done in California; if they fail, they die. It obviously raises major social, ethical and political issues. The logic of explicit rationing is that rationing becomes explicit and forced into the open.

Luke Zander (General Practitioner, London) Would you like to make a comment about the possible role that we, as professionals, have in encouraging Government to maintain data collection, processing and distribution systems?

Professor Maynard This is a disaster. The Korner information system has not come on stream and the Government is really lying low about why this is so. Hence they have very little routine hospital data. The Resource Management Initiative reported that the system has been very poor in the six sites where it was actually used. It is possible that the reform of the NHS has committed about £300 million to information technology, and the fear is that this will not produce much information which is useful for evaluation, let alone patient management. It is very depressing.

Rupert Fawdry (Obstetrician, Milton Keynes) As somebody who takes an interest in information technology and computers, it is particularly sad to see the speed at which changes in the NHS are being made. The technology is not there and money is being thrown straight onto a bonfire. Bath has just got a £4 million computer system that is out of date technologically and is not going to help us. Until the technology has actually moved on to the next stage and can be supportive to individual patient care, we are not going to get data out in a cost–benefit way.

Professor Maynard All I can say is that when the Public Accounts Committee gets round to looking at it, there are going to be very vigorous expressions of interest. If the figures of about £300 million are right, it is an enormous amount of money to have been spent, given the funding of the NHS for patient care.

Renata Dharmisena (Head of Midwifery Education, St Leonards-on-Sea) We should look at health costs as an investment just as we should be looking at costs in education and training. The term, cost, in itself has a negative connotation. Health costs invested in individuals means investing in economic units; each one of us contributes to the wealth of this country and if you can improve health, you can return people to a state of economic viability, contributing yet more wealth to society.

Professor Maynard This is what we are trying to do, but the emphasis must be on being very careful about how you measure the benefits from the investment. If you measure them in terms of productivity and other issues that you are raising, there are major problems. Since women are paid less than men for a variety of social reasons, if you take the investment approach you would not invest as much in women as you would in men. People over 65 are not going to take much part in the labour force. When attempting to measure the benefits from your investment you have to be extremely careful not to use financial measures which would bias your investment.

3

Legal influences on clinical practice

Robert Dingwall

In legal terms, the delivery of babies is one of the most complicated areas of medical practice. Care providers have a uniquely powerful monopoly over the right to assist a woman in childbirth, while being exceptionally vulnerable to negligence litigation if anything goes wrong. Childbirth is the only area of health care where most clinical actions affect two potential plaintiffs at the same time. This dual liability, to mother and child, accounts for much of the legal complexity. The professionals have to strike a delicate balance between the interests of mothers and their babies, when only the former group has the resources and ability to articulate and press its claims. At the same time, there is a more general societal interest in the health and well-being of children, which is expressed in some of the legal forms of professional accountability and which may represent a conflicting consideration in any particular case. This tension runs from the moment of conception to the end of a child's period of dependency. It is focused on a great debate of principle over the relative priority to attach to parental rights to autonomy and privacy and the children's rights to protection from harm and the stimulation of their human potential. Since children cannot act as advocates on their own behalf, these rights can only be made real by interventions which compromise the rights of their parents.

In a brief review, it is not possible to do justice to all the issues involved and this paper will focus on two examples – the regulation of birth attendants and the effects of tort liability. However, it is important not to detach these cases from their wider context, and to neglect the extent to which professionals are actually being asked to produce practical resolutions of eternally debatable questions in social and political philosophy.

31

A PROFESSIONAL MONOPOLY[1-3]

Until April 1910, assistance in the delivery of babies was a free market. Anybody could set themselves up as a birth attendant. They were not required to satisfy any licensing body or to conform to any professional discipline, although, of course, they always remained subject to the general criminal and civil law. Midwifery had become a mandatory part of basic medical education in 1879 and any practitioner registered after that could at least pretend to some formal training. Doctors, however, performed only a small proportion of the deliveries carried out in Britain. By far the largest proportion were carried out by midwives, the majority of whom had no formal preparation for the work and a significant minority of whom were poor, aged, dirty or illiterate. With the passage of the Midwives Act 1902, though, it became unlawful for anyone to deliver babies 'habitually and for gain' other than a licensed medical practitioner, a woman working under the supervision of such a practitioner or a woman whose name had been entered on the roll of the Central Midwives Board, either by virtue of some certificate or from being of good character and in *bona fide* practice for one year prior to April 1905. This definition contained a number of loopholes, which allowed a measure of unlicensed practice to continue, with some collusion from individual doctors, but it was progressively tightened by subsequent Acts in 1926, 1936, 1951 and 1979. The current legislation, the Nurses, Midwives and Health Visitors Act 1979, baldly states that: 'A person other than a registered midwife or a registered medical practitioner shall not attend a woman in childbirth.'

The only defence, covering people like taxi drivers, ambulance crews and police officers acting as Good Samaritans, is that the delivery was performed by an unlicensed person as a matter of 'sudden and urgent necessity'. The qualified exemption for women practising under the supervision of a medical practitioner has now been explicitly limited to students of medicine and midwifery attending courses recognized by their licensing boards.

In medicolegal terms, this is a very unusual state of affairs. People are generally free to choose between seeking or not seeking treatment for health care problems. If they want to obtain treatment, they have considerable discretion whether to use self-medication, to consult friends or relatives informally, to visit an unregistered practitioner of some sort or to attend a licensed medical practitioner. While there are important legal disadvantages to the provision of health care by unregistered practitioners, there is nothing which actually bars them from practice. The advantages of the registered practitioner do not rest on a legally-backed monopoly of the right to provide diagnosis, advice or treatment. Why is obstetrics or midwifery different?

The main accounts of the development of midwifery licensing from the 1870s onwards tend to present this as the result of a convergence of occupational, gender and philanthropic interests. Donnison[4] suggests five distinct constituencies of support:

(1)   Women seeking to create a high status occupation complementary to the medical profession; this group eventually split as some gained access to that profession while others held out for their ideal of a highly educated independent practitioner;

(2)   Women concerned to establish a low-cost alternative to doctors for the poor;

(3)   Male obstetricians who wanted a low-cost subordinate dealing with routine cases and poorer patients, shutting out general practitioners from the market for middle-class deliveries by denying them opportunities to gain experience of this work;

(4)   General practitioners themselves seeking to use regulation as a way of controlling or suppressing cut-price competition;

(5)   Lady nurses around Mrs Bedford Fenwick who hoped to use midwifery licensing as a stalking horse for the registration of general nurses.

In almost all of these groups it is very hard to disentangle consideration of self-interest and public good.

However, Donnison's work lies within a particular tradition in the study of occupational development which tends to emphasize *demand* factors in the establishment of professional monopolies. It needs to be complemented by some consideration of the *supply* of regulation, of the state's response. At any time, there are always more occupations that would like licensure and its special legal protections than any state will consider it appropriate to endorse. An understanding of the reasons why, after several decades of resistance, the government acted in 1900 to prepare a Bill for the licensing of midwives may help us to understand the objectives of closing this particular market and their implications for current practice.

Unfortunately, the government's motives for initiating the process of market closure have not attracted much interest from historians. Donnison notes that the Midwives Bill was introduced into the middle of the debate on National Efficiency, sparked off by General J.F. Maurice's revelations about the poor health of recruits to the army during the Boer War, which had profound consequences for the massive development of policy on infant welfare under the 1906–11 Liberal Government. However, the commitment to legislation predates the publication of Maurice's articles so their impact cannot explain the government's original initiative. There had, though, been a number of developments in the late 1890s, like the Infant Life Preservation Act 1897, which had strengthened the powers of local authorities to supervise fostering and child-minding with the objective of reducing the abuses of baby farming. The welfare of babies and children had already been raised as an issue before it became transformed by the arguments over National Efficiency. Certainly, there can be little doubt that the vigour with which the Midwives Act was administered in many areas owed a good deal to the heightened concern about the quality of social reproduction revealed by the military failures of the Boer War and the commercial failures of the long economic recession of the 1880s and 1890s. Britain was faced with active competition from other imperial and industrial powers whose success was thought to owe much to their more deliberate attention to the welfare of their peoples and, in particular, to the conditions under which the next generation was born and raised.

The importance of this is that the monopoly must be regarded as something which was motivated by concerns for child protection as much as for the welfare of mothers. This is not to say that mothers were unimportant, merely that their well-being was important only because they were mothers and that physical unfitness might compromise their willingness to bear children and to contribute actively to their upbringing. It is part of an expression of the view that the health of children is not a purely private interest, but one in which the community as a whole has a stake. By creating the monopoly, health care providers became agents of the community, subject to obligations which could, ultimately, override the wishes of their clients, even in the course of a private transaction. This is a dimension of practice which has been neglected in many recent debates, or evaded by the simplistic assertion that parents in general, or mothers in particular, are the best judges of their children's interests. The whole point of a division of labour is to reflect the impossibility in a modern society of everyone being an expert on everything and, in this sense at least, professionals do have to, on occasion, know better. Monopolies, such as the one discussed here, reflect the inability of the market to deliver information to consumers in circumstances which are highly consequential to their 'health ... fortune ... life and reputation'[5]. In this case, of course, the problem is compounded by the limitations on the capacity of babies to act as rational decision-makers! Contemporary transactions between women and their birth attendants are not purely private matters.

TORT LIABILITY

The fact that birth attendants may have obligations to a community beyond the immediate participants in the birth process does not, of course, mean that they have no obligations to mothers and their children. One of the most fundamental of these is the duty of care under the common law of tort. This is one of the oldest methods of holding professionals accountable for their actions, with cases against medical practitioners dating back to the fourteenth century. The basis of a tort action for negligence is the assumption that all members of a society have a duty to behave with reasonable care in their dealings with each other. If I fail in this duty and this has the consequence of causing you some injury, then you are entitled to seek compensation from me for any resulting economic losses and for the general upset which you have experienced. Looked at another way, the fact that I may have to compensate you creates an incentive for me to take care. I must assess whether the likely benefits from a risky course of action are likely to be outweighed by the potential losses which I may suffer if it goes wrong and I have to compensate you for some injury. My loss may also send a signal to others like me about the possible consequences of actions of this sort and thereby affect their decision-making.

Until 1948, both doctors and midwives were, in the main, individually liable for their actions. If something went wrong, they could be sued as individuals and would be liable to pay compensation from their own pockets. In practice, only doctors would have had sufficient resources to be worth suing and they developed a form of insurance against this risk with the establishment of bodies like the Medical Defence Union, the Medical Protection Society and the Medical and Dental Defence Union of Scotland. After 1948, all National Health Service midwives became covered by the vicarious liability of their employer. This is a form of liability where an employer takes responsibility for the actions of employees within the scope of their employment. It is designed partly to ensure that victims of injury can recover compensation from someone who has a deeper pocket and is better able to provide the necessary resources, and partly to discourage employers from putting their staff in positions where they will knowingly take risks rather than incur sanctions from managers or supervisors. Since that time, any negligence by an NHS midwife has resulted in an action against her employing authority, which has a theoretical right to join her in the action as an individual and to attempt to recover its losses from her. As far as I can ascertain, this right has never been exercised, although it might attract the interest of some hard-nosed Trust managers.

The medical profession, however, thought that it was important that they should continue to have an explicit influence over the way litigation was handled. They feared that NHS authorities might handle cases on a simple economic basis and that some claims might be settled purely because it was cheaper to pay than to fight. Where a doctor's professional reputation was at stake, such a policy could have considerable personal costs, in that a settlement, even without an admission of liability, was likely to damage his or her standing with patients or peers. At a rather later point, the fear was also expressed that health authorities might be less willing to pursue what were essentially test cases for a new technique or mode of practice, where the costs of the individual action might be quite disproportionate to the losses alleged, encouraging settlement, but where the implications for the profession as a whole might be considerable. From 1954 until 1990, then, liability was shared between health authorities and employed doctors (GPs as independent contractors always remained individually liable). However, this system broke down under pressures from the rising costs and numbers of negligence actions in the 1980s and was replaced by a form of employer's liability. Although there are some technical differences, all NHS birth attendants are now covered by essentially the same legal arrangements, with the major costs falling on their employers, in the latest incarnation of the scheme, provider units and NHS Trusts.

The growth in litigation is thought by many to have had a disproportionate effect on the practice of obstetrics. In reality, the picture is a good deal more complicated than simple statistics might suggest and there are some serious questions about the interpretation of the profession's response. There is also an argument that the problem has been made worse rather than better by the Department of Health's latest version of NHS Indemnity.

It is not disputed that obstetrics and gynaecology cases contribute a significant proportion of the negligence cases brought against the NHS. In a study of the 470 closed claims traceable against District Health Authorities in the Oxford Region between 1974 and 1988, Paul Fenn and I found that 22% of the claims originated from this area. However, they represented only 16.7% of the successful claims and 8.8% of the total loss to the NHS. For this Region in this period, claims had a lower than average success rate and were concluded with relatively small payments. As it happens, the series did not include any major brain-damaged baby cases. However, this finding is not inconsistent with the indications that cases of this kind were being opened at a rate of 50–100 per year nationally throughout this period and that the mean duration was 6.7 years[6,7]. Even if the recent change in the legal aid rules leads to an increase in the base rate to 200 cases a year, this would still only be one per district per year. Since the success rate seems to be around 25–30%[7–9], this suggests that the typical district will only be hit with a big payout once every four years and is unlikely to be able to predict its liability any more precisely. With the liability being transferred to provider units and Trusts, of course, its impact is likely to be even more erratic. This is not to be dismissive of the problem: the Medical Protection Society has estimated that obstetric cases make up 30% of the total loss of the profession's liability carriers[6]. However, a sense of perspective is important: big obstetric cases are not an everyday phenomenon, although they can have major implications for defendants when they do occur.

How can this be reconciled with the various alarums and excursions which have emanated from the obstetric fraternity? Is litigation really having a big effect on the practice of obstetrics and the recruitment to the specialty? Three points seem important here. The first is that, with the exception of the present temporary blip as a result of changes in legal aid rules, there is no evidence that obstetrics has had a significantly different experience from the rest of the medical profession. Indeed, if anything, its share of the total volume of negligence litigation may have declined slightly in the 1980s[7]. As has been pointed out elsewhere, most professions experienced an upsurge in negligence litigation in the 1980s and it seems likely that any explanation of the trend will involve reference to factors that are not exclusive to the provision of health care. Secondly, there is no convincing evidence that litigation has played more than a minor role in changing clinical practice.

Caesarean section rates have increased world-wide, regardless of the litigation experience of different countries and the survey evidence from the USA is inconclusive (see Figure 1)[10]. Most of the findings can be as well explained by the changing economic context of American practice[11]. Finally, the argument that it is having a deterrent effect on recruitment seems inconsistent with what is known about the process of career choice and the variety of influences which determine the pursuit of one track rather than another[12]. To the extent that there are problems in recruitment to obstetrics, they may have more to do with the gloomy comments of senior figures than the actual experience of the specialty.

It may, then, be more important to understand what people are doing with the rhetoric of legal obligation and, in particular, the way in which this can form a dimension of struggles for control of the delivery process, where real issues of gender and occupational politics can be concealed in an apparently technical language. To these must now be added the concerns of unit or Trust managements, engaged in what is likely to be a futile effort to control their liability to the swingeing

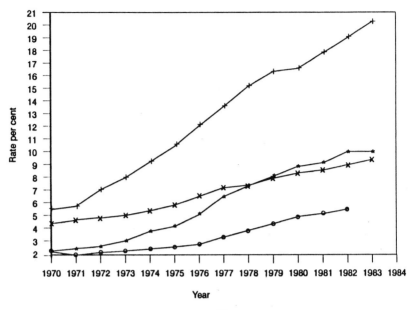

Figure 1 Caesarean section rates 1970–83[10]: (+ = USA; × = England and Wales; * = Norway, and ○ = The Netherlands)

penalties that will be imposed by the Department of Health indemnity scheme. It must also be noted that it is unlikely that any one unit or Trust will be happy to risk the costs of fighting the major test case on the causation of cerebral palsy that is now clearly necessary. The individually rational action of settling a case rather than risking the extra costs of fighting and losing can easily produce a collectively irrational result. One can only look forward to confusion and disarray in the immediate future.

Obstetrics and midwifery are always liable to be legally problematic areas of practice with the complexities of their dual accountability to mothers and babies and the high emotions which attach to this great moment in the lives of women and their partners. Of course every parent wants a perfect baby but nature does not always oblige. However, a more stoic acceptance of these realities by the professionals involved might lead both to an attempt to explain the dilemmas of their practice and to focus the issues in their proper domain of moral debate. How do we protect children without tyrannizing women? Should the care of handicapped children rest on a legal lottery or become a matter of collective responsibility at a more generous level than the meagre provisions of social security? Let us not blame the professionals for the terms we have imposed on them.

ACKNOWLEDGEMENTS

The section on Tort Liability draws extensively on work conducted in collaboration with Paul Fenn at the Centre for Socio-Legal Studies, University of Oxford, and supported by funding from the economic and Social Research Council, Oxford Regional Health Authority and Oxfordshire District Health Authority.

REFERENCES

1. Dingwall, R., Rafferty, A.M. and Webster, C. (1988). *An Introduction to the Social History of Nursing*, pp. 145–72. (London: Routledge)
2. Eekelaar, J.M. and Dingwall, R. (1984). Some legal issues in obstetric practice. *J. Social Welfare Law*, 258–70
3. Dingwall, R. and Fenn, P. (1987). 'A respectable profession?' Sociological and economic perspectives on the regulation of professional services. *Int. Rev. Law and Econ.*, 7, 51–64
4. Donnison, J. (1977). *Midwives and Medical Men*. (London: Heinemann)
5. Smith, A. (1976). (First published 1776). *An Inquiry into the Nature and Causes of the Wealth of Nations*. (Chicago: University of Chicago Press)
6. Acheson, D. (1991). Law suit crisis poses threat to obstetric care. *Hospital Doctor*, C11, 12
7. Capstick, J.B. and Edwards, P.J. (1990). Medicine and the law: Trends in obstetric malpractice claims. *Lancet*, 336, 931–2
8. Dingwall, R. and Fenn, P. (1991). Risk management in the National Health Service: Who needs it? *Int. J. Risk and Safety in Med.*, 2, 91–106
9. Hawkins, C. and Patterson, I. (1987). Medicolegal audit in the West Midlands Region: Analysis of 100 cases. *Br. Med. J.*, 295, 1533–6
10. Macfarlane and Mugford (1986). An epidemic of Caesareans. *J. Matern. Child Health*, 11, 38–42
11. Quam, L., Dingwall, R. and Fenn, P. (1988). Medical malpractice claims in obstetrics and gynaecology: Comparisons between the United States and Britain. *Br. J. Obstet. Gynaecol.*, 95, 454–61

4

The development of health care policies

Chris Ham

I would like to start with two caveats. The first is that I am not a specialist on maternity care issues. I have been asked to add a policy dimension to what has been said so far in order to provide the context for the rest of the conference and so will use some maternity care examples to illustrate my argument. The second caveat is that I shall be specifically discussing health care policies and will not be commenting on broader social policies and developments in welfare generally. This is not because I consider these wider issues to be unimportant, it is simply because of the space available.

If we are trying to understand the development of health care policies, then we must do so at four levels[1]. Firstly there is the national dimension, that is, the way in which the Department of Health formulates policies for health care, including its relationship with pressure groups and the health care professions. Secondly there is the local dimension, or the development of policies within district health authorities. Health authorities play an important part in planning and managing health services and this includes their new role as purchasers under the NHS reforms. Thirdly, there is the link between national and local levels. This draws our attention to the implementation of health care policies, and, in some cases, the non-implementation of these policies. Finally, there is the point at which doctors and nurses actually deliver services to patients. This is the last link in the policy chain and in a professionalized service such as the NHS it is particularly important because of the large measure of discretion professionals have in shaping how policies are implemented in practice.

THE NATIONAL DIMENSION

To begin with the national policy-making process, one of the ideas currently in vogue in the policy analysis literature is that of policy communities. A policy community is a cluster of organizations and agencies concerned with a particular area of government activity. Each community is centred on a Government department. The term 'community' is meant to signify the close relationships and shared priorities that often develop between Government departments and outside interests[2]. This is not to say that there is always agreement between the members of a policy community but simply that there is a common interest in the policies or services concerned. As a consequence, there is often a wish to see these services receive higher priority within Government as a whole even if there are different views on how the budget should be divided up.

In the case of the Department of Health, the health policy community is made up of the Department itself and a range of organizations interested in its work and concerned to influence policies for health services. These include pressure groups representing both patients on the one hand and professional or provider interests on the other; these include the Maternity Alliance, the National Childbirth Trust, and the Association for the Improvement of Maternity Services as well as medical, nursing and midwifery organizations. The funding that the Government provides to support patient and consumer organizations is an illustration of the importance of the idea of the policy community. On the face of it, it seems rather odd that Government should provide financial support to agencies which then act to put pressure on the Government. This occurs because it helps the Department of Health to have pressure from outside organizations in its own discussions with the Treasury for funding for health services.

Next is Parliament, including both individual Members and, increasingly, the Select Committees. Both the Social Services Committee and the Public Accounts Committee have turned their attention to maternity issues and their influence has become increasingly apparent over the years.

A further source of influence is the mass media. Both radio and TV have an important role to play in getting issues onto the crowded health policy agenda. In some cases they go beyond this to take on a campaigning role on particular issues.

Surrounding the Department of Health is the official advisory machinery. This comprises committees, groups and working parties which advise the Department on health care policy. A good example would be the Maternity Services Advisory Committee.

Finally the role of Health Authorities should be considered. They are responsible not just for implementing health care policy but also for influencing its formulation at national level. This they do both through individual managers and chairmen contributing to national policy development and through the work of the National Association of Health Authorities and Trusts.

Within the health policy community, what often happens is that sub-communities develop around particular issues. These sub-communities bring together those organizations and individuals interested in specific policies such as those concerning alcohol, care of elderly people and maternity services. Outside agencies are drawn towards those parts of the Department that deal with their area of interest. The people concerned tend to know each other well and have a good deal of informal as well as formal contact.

To introduce another piece of jargon, the relationships that then develop can be likened to *iron triangles* or *issue networks*. Iron triangles exist when there are firm, stable relationships between a few key interests. A study of policies for elderly people found that there was an iron triangle comprising DHSS officials, the Royal College of Nursing and the British Geriatrics Society, and a few leading doctors and nurses[3]. There was wider consultation with other organizations but the crucial early decisions in this case involved a few key organizations and individuals.

Issue networks are much more fluid and flexible. They do not involve fixed, stable relationships. They do allow greater scope for a range of individuals and groups to shape what goes on. I have not found an example in the research literature of how policies for maternity services are formulated but these ideas may be helpful in our discussions at this conference.

THE LOCAL DIMENSION

At the second level of the policy-making process, the district health authority, a similar sort of analysis can be applied. Not only is there a national health policy community centred on the Department of Health but there is also a series of local health policy communities based on individual health districts. As with the Department of Health, health authorities are surrounded by a number of groups in their localities. These groups are interested in health care and seek to influence the decisions of health authorities. The organizations concerned include local pressure groups (for example the Community Health Council), Members of Parliament and local politicians, press and radio, advisory machinery (especially professional advisory machinery) and other health authorities, such as the regional health authority and family health services authority.

The district health authority itself includes the chairman, the non-executive members and managers. Describing the local health policy community in this way gives the appearance of a relatively open, democratic and pluralistic process. Of course, it is not quite like that. All the research evidence suggests that within health authorities themselves, the key players are usually the chairman and general manager with non-executive members in a relatively marginal position.

In turn, the chairman and general manager are not free agents. They operate in the context of a national service in which all of their money comes from the Treasury. In addition, the Department of Health has issued increasingly detailed national and regional guidance which has limited the freedom of manoeuvre of district health authorities. Among the local groups and interests, some are clearly more powerful than others. Very often, it is the views of local professional groups which are most important. These views provide the driving force in the NHS and on most issues are a good deal more powerful than the views of the Community Health Council and local voluntary groups[4].

NATIONAL AND LOCAL LINKS

The third level is the link between national and local policy-making, often referred to as the implementation process. The point to emphasize here is that the relationship between the Department of Health and health authorities is not cast in stone. Looking back over the history of the NHS, the extent of national involvement in local affairs has varied between different periods. The balance of power and influence has swung back and forth like a pendulum and what we are now experiencing is a period of very strong central control with the Department of Health very much in the driving seat.

The Department uses a range of instruments to ensure that national policies are taken seriously by district health authorities. Of these instruments, the planning and review process is the most important. Following the NHS reforms, this is still developing, but in essence it involves the chief executive of the NHS issuing guidelines on priorities to health authorities. Authorities then prepare plans in the light of national guidelines and the NHS Management Executive agrees a corporate contract with each regional health authority. This sets out how regions will take forward their services in the next 12 months. In turn, regional health authorities agree corporate contracts with district health authorities and the success or failure of authorities in achieving their objectives is checked through the review process. This culminates in the annual review meeting between different tiers of management.

Despite these arrangements, there is still no guarantee that national policies will be implemented at a local level, but the combination of national guidelines, corporate contracts and review meetings provides an important and powerful instrument for ensuring much greater consistency between health authorities with national policies. In this context, given the theme of this volume, it is relevant to note that maternity services were one of only two national service priorities for 1991–2 singled out by Duncan Nichol when he wrote to health authorities last July. I am sure that one of the reasons for that was the series of critical reports produced by the Social Services Committee and, particularly, the Public Accounts Committee in recent years. These reports have helped to give maternity services a higher place on a crowded national policy agenda.

THE POINT OF DELIVERY

The fourth level is concerned with the way in which policies are carried into practice by doctors, nurses and other staff. This is especially important in a professionalized service like health care because policies rarely specify in detail what should be done. There is also a good deal of diversity between different areas because professionals will have their own views on what is appropriate in terms of service provision. Indeed, this point could be put more strongly in that policy in the health services often originates through professional practices. Innovations often emerge from professional practice and are then picked up and disseminated along professional networks. Policy-makers at a district, regional or national level have to respond to professionally driven service changes rather than professionals having to respond to politically driven service changes. To put the point rather differently, policy development is both bottom-up and top-down and we need to be aware of this in trying to understand how policies are made and in seeking to influence these policies.

INFLUENCES ON POLICY-MAKING

In the light of this it should be clear that there are a number of key points at which policies emerge and are shaped. It is also the case that policy-making is in part a rational process spurred on by facts, information and argument, and in part it is a political process in which what happens owes more to the power of different groups than to any rational analysis of what should happen. This means that for the most part the pressure groups and organizations representing professional views carry more weight than the groups representing patients and service users. As the example of the iron triangle for elderly people illustrated, it was doctors, nurses and their professional organizations which were closely involved in policy-making, not Age Concern and other user-based agencies.

To emphasize the political nature of the policy-making process is not to argue that research and information have no influence. Clearly they do in some cases. The point is that research needs to be hitched to a political wagon before it really enters the policy arena. That is why the work of the Public Accounts Committee and the Social Services Committee has been important in the maternity services field in recent years. In providing a voice with which to articulate some of the issues emerging from the professional and research world, these committees have played an important role in the development of thinking and policy.

There is no direct correlation between the quality of research and ideas and the impact they have on policy. One only has to compare the minimal impact of the Black Report on inequalities in health with the powerful influence of, say, Alain Enthoven's ideas on the NHS reforms, to appreciate this point. Comprehensively documented analysis will have no influence if it is born into a hostile political environment. Equally, relatively modest ideas can be important if they are timely and coincide with developments on the political agenda.

It is also worth adding that researchers do not always help their own cause by the way research results are presented. All of my experience tells me that politicians and civil servants are such busy people that they need research results to be presented clearly and attractively. In this sense, researchers need to be skilful advocates themselves, actively promoting their findings and not assuming that rigorous research producing new evidence will speak for itself.

IMPACT OF NHS REFORMS

I have never been one of those who has argued that the reforms will undermine the basic principles of the NHS and lead to privatization through the back door. There are some good things in the reforms and some bad things. The real test comes as they are implemented when we see if the positive features can outweigh the negative.

From a policy perspective, the most important change is the separation of purchaser and provider roles. Health authorities have been given the responsibility of assessing the population's need for health care and of purchasing health care services. This means that in future those organizations and interests making claims for extra resources will have to justify these claims to a body no longer so close to professional and provider interests. Health authorities will be able to take a more detached and independent view of needs and priorities. That will not involve dramatic or rapid changes in service provision but it could strengthen the position of public health doctors, health economists and managers in purchasing roles, and it could open up new channels for patient and community groups to influence policy. It will also give GPs a greater say both through the fund-holding scheme and through the dialogue now developing between district health authorities and GPs. What this means is that hospital doctors, nurses and midwives will be much more on the defensive as purchasers ask some tough questions about the costs and benefits of the services provided.

This will not only affect maternity care; it will apply across the whole range of service provision. It will mean that those claims supported by hard evidence of benefits will be easier to substantiate than those that are not. Health authorities as purchasers will be looking for best buys and the contracts they negotiate with providers will make more visible and transparent what should be provided. As such, these contracts provide an important new mechanism for setting standards. These standards are likely to reflect both good professional practice and patients' needs and preferences.

None of this will happen if we bury our heads in the sand and hope the reforms will go away. They are here to stay and people who are prepared to take advantage of new opportunities will find that there is scope for bringing about improvements in services that have long been argued for.

REFERENCES

1. Ham, C.J. (1985). *Health Policy in Britain,* 2nd edn. (London: Macmillan)
2. Richardson, J.J. and Jordan, A.G. (1979). *Governing Under Pressure.* (Oxford: Martin Robertson)
3. Haywood, S. and Hunter, D.A. (1982). Consultative processes in health policy in the United Kingdom: a view from the centre. *Public Administration,* **69,** 143–62
4. Ham, C.J. (1986). *Managing Health Services.* (Bristol: School for Advanced Urban Studies, University of Bristol)

General discussion I

Professor Geoffrey Chamberlain (Obstetrician, London) The first part of Professor Dingwall's presentation focused on how we got into the present position of law about a woman having a baby. In the second part, he talked about the complex business of litigation and its effect on the profession, and asked three questions:

(1) Has obstetrics had a greater onslaught of cases than the rest of the profession? The Medical Protection Society and Medical Defence Union who used to represent 95% of the doctors up to 1990 have published data on this showing obstetric cases to be one-third up on other specialties. It often takes 5–10 years for a case to come to fruition, but data on claims opened as well as cases settled indicate that we are at much greater risk.

(2) Has it affected practice? Using the argument about Caesarean section rates, in the data he presented there were different rates in the two countries (USA and UK) with more legal problems than in those countries without Caesarean sections have been affected by medicolegal fears.

(3) Has it affected recruitment? This is a hard question to answer. We have some data at the Royal College of Obstetricians and Gynaecologists that show it has. We now are down to barely replacement levels among senior house officers coming through to be the Registrars and Senior Registrars of the future. This is something we have not seen before. Obstetricians are retiring earlier so that our mean retirement age is now down from 63 to 58 years. Although I do not like quoting other countries, the American College of Obstetricians and Gynecologists has published a survey recently showing that 25% of obstetricians have either stopped or cut back doing obstetrics and are doing gynaecology only. This is a précis of the data showing that the legal explosion has affected the profession.

Professor Robert Dingwall (Sociologist, Nottingham) If I can comment on these three specific points. The first is about the share of claims against the medical profession represented by obstetrics. It is clearly a specialty which accounts for a very large proportion of the claims, compared with orthopaedics which figures much less prominently, but which can also lead to very costly cases. However, it is not the case that obstetrics is way out of line when looking at closed and open claims. The comment I made was about the share of claims in a database held by Capsticks (a firm of solicitors in south-west London) on claims opened, which does not suggest that although obstetrics is a high-risk specialty, the risk has not increased disproportionately during the 1980s.

The second point is about the data on the Caesarean section rates. The point here is that although the levels may be higher in absolute terms, in countries with a higher rate of litigation the important thing is that the rate of increase is comparable in all four countries, which suggests that it is driven by very much the same technical considerations: the change in the risk–benefit ratio of the procedure, and the estimate of the desirability of repeat Caesarean sections.

The third point referred to factors influencing recruitment. I think there are a variety of reasons why obstetrics is an area of medicine with diminishing attractiveness. On the specific point of the American surveys, what you can see is that the areas where people are moving out of obstetric practice are also the areas where obstetric practices are essentially unprofitable. They are ageing, sparsely settled communities. The point to make is that in America, medicine is very responsive to market forces and market forces, quite aside from the costs of malpractice insurance and the frequency of suing, are making obstetrics economically unattractive in certain parts of the country. That is the way their system works.

Mr Stanley Simmons (President, Royal College of Obstetricians and Gynaecologists) There has been a tremendous change in the litigation scene in the last 2–3 years. As an example, we had a meeting at the RCOG about a month ago with 200 people attending, mostly consultants. We asked the question: 'How many had been the subject of litigation?' and virtually every hand in the room went up. We then asked how many had been settled out of court and virtually all those hands went up again. So it is very difficult to get accurate figures through cases that come to court. They are hidden by the fact that the great majority are being settled out of court.

The impact on recruitment is extremely difficult to analyse, but I do think the way in which consultants behave, as a reaction to medicolegal complaints, particularly in terms of retiring early, has a profound effect on young people. They see dissatisfied seniors but it is very difficult to maintain a positive outlook when you know it is virtually certain you

50

are going to be involved in litigation within your lifetime, perhaps many times. This is having a very significant effect on the specialty and it is something we must continue to try to grapple with.

It does seem a particularly uncivilized way to behave towards brain-damaged infants and their families that whether or not they gain extra financial support depends entirely on the tort system of litigation; this is something we should continue to try to change.

Doris Shaw (Midwife, USA) The State of West Virginia has recently passed legislation which greatly limits the tort system. After spending $25 million, not one child has been benefited so far. The State of New York also is considering changing its medicolegal system. I do not think it will go through but they consider that in the first year it will cost the State $185 million. Aside from that, the State of New York spent $3.5 million to look at the rate of medical malpractice suits occurring in the State. They found that for every case that was brought to light there were nine clear-cut cases of medical malpractice that never saw the light of day. It is important that we ask professionals to look at their practice and see what could be avoided that would make maternal and infant outcome better.

Jilly Rosser (Institute of Child Health, Bristol) Litigation affects midwives as well as obstetricians. Talking to midwives around the country, it seems that fear of litigation has had a very strong influence on midwives' practice. This may not influence Caesarean section rates, but it will intrude upon the flexibility of midwifery care and on other important things. It is not fear of litigation from the mother and the baby, it is fear of litigation from within their own profession and from their own statutory bodies. It is an entirely different picture but it has a very strong influence.

Richard Porter (Obstetrician, Bath) Professor Dingwall raised the possibility that the employer might choose to take the part of the plaintiff or with the damaged child, against the professional. Our Health Authority looked into this and guidance from the Department was that this was wholly contrary to the concept of Crown Indemnity. That statement was made last year; it may be that since the new NHS has come in, things have changed.

Chris Ham mentioned the extent to which much of the reorganization is introducing more authoritarian direction rather than the downward delegation of power and responsibility that it was widely advertized as doing. We have seen other issues in the area of contracts where questions have been raised about what the Department of Health actually meant by a contract and what could legally be done under the condition of contracts. The Department's answer has been that when problems come up, they simply will not let it happen.

The situation here is exactly the same, in that legally there is nothing to prevent an employer from bringing an employee into an action and then seeking to recover the costs from them. The only thing restraining them is the directive from the Department of Health, that this was not within the spirit of what was intended by the re-disorganization. In the same way, various things which might happen under the contractual regime are dealt with in a similarly arbitrary fashion. I do think that the increase in the exercise of arbitrary power by the Department of Health as a result of this re-disorganization is something which we should not lose sight of lightly.

Iain Chalmers (National Perinatal Epidemiology Unit, Oxford) I want to challenge Chris Ham's suggestion that researchers are the right people to learn how to produce their results in an attractive way for people who have to take decisions on the basis of that research. I think that it is unreasonable to expect people to have skills across the whole range of the development and application of new therapies, from basic research to clinical trials to dissemination to application. It is as though one required drug companies to sack all their promotional people and rely on the research workers in those companies actually to communicate the results of that research.

They do have a duty however to write up their research. It was shown very clearly in a recent copy of *The Lancet* that they are not doing this. *The Lancet* showed that not only do large quantities of research not get written up at all, but in addition, the research which is reported has more statistically significant results that interest the investigators than the research that does not get written up.

Professor Chris Ham I have a good deal of sympathy with Iain Chalmer's question although I think it is not quite as clear-cut. Some researchers are already good advocates for their research results, seeing that as a priority, and they put a lot of effort into the dissemination of their findings. I would like to see more of that. In a sense, I would like to throw the question back, if researchers do not give more priority to it, who will? Would you be appointing a marketing manager to your unit who will go out and sell your ideas? I do not say this as a flippant comment; if we are serious about it, then that is what we ought to be doing, and if the grant-givers will also see it as having a high priority, they will provide the necessary resources.

Mary Newburn (National Childbirth Trust) I have a linked comment about both papers. Professor Dingwall said that he thinks professionals do sometimes know best; the question I would ask is, which professionals? Are they the obstetricians, midwives or researchers or any of the other professionals? I think very often some of the issues that service users want to raise not only concern their own experience of the way in which care is provided, but relate to the actual content of that care. I think that kind of input is sometimes not taken proper account of.

The politics of policy-making is very important but users are not very powerful players in this particular political area. Very largely we do not have resources, not only because we are not budget holders in terms of providing services, but because our own resources within our organizations are very slender. We simply do not have the staff to do the lobbying needed. This was brought home to me recently in the Public Accounts Committee Report, following the National Audit Office Report, both of which are extremely important documents. But there are few user organizations that are quoted and the issues that are important to them are also sparse. This is not because we do not think the issues are important, it is because we have not got large bodies of administrators, researchers and politicians working for us to actually get the issues that we want raised in the public arena.

Sarah Roach (Midwife, Southampton) I think we have to shed our political naivety and use important bodies, such as the Public Accounts Committee, which are now commenting increasingly on professional issues. There has been an extremely useful comment recently about the proper utilization of midwives' skills from the Public Accounts Committee, but also we need to learn how to feed information into this body. We have not got many resources, but unless we do this, we will not be acting in the public interest in this hard-nosed economic climate. The pressure groups and professionals must stand alongside each other in the public interest or the public will be immensely the poorer.

Marion Hall (Obstetrician, Aberdeen) I want to comment on the question of GPs as purchasers. It really had not occurred to me until this meeting that while the midwives are providers, purely and strictly, GPs in the new NHS Act are both purchasers and providers. If there were a contest between GPs and midwives, about who is going to provide the primary care for pregnant women, the GP in his quasi-purchaser role has an unfair advantage over the midwife. I do not wish to set this up as though there were a conflict because in fact, GPs and midwives usually collaborate very happily. It is an important issue however that the new NHS

Act does not really acknowledge the fact that the GP is not always entirely disinterested from the point of view of professional power.

Irene Hinchelwood (East Hertfordshire Health Authority) On our Health Authority, we consider that we have both nursing and medical professionals putting their points of view and we also have a Community Health Council observer who comes to our meetings. We are trying to consider all opinions.

One of the problems is that the public conception of the new NHS Act is that everything is going to happen right away. It has now passed the starting time and the public expects to see great changes, but the health authorities do not yet have freedom of action because we must put our contracts where they have been placed in the past. We hope that we will be able to change the balance of spending over the years, but one of the things that bothers me is how we are going to monitor the quality of care.

Wendy Savage (Obstetrician, Royal London Hospital) Since research has had so little effect on Government policy so far, what makes us think that the provider/purchaser money oriented relationship will make any difference? It is depressing that we have an NHS reorganization forced upon us against the will of the people and that we have now health authorities in which there is no representation of professionals who actually know what goes on from the shop floor, with an increasing pressure for money to be raised by health authorities for facilities the Government should be providing with the money we give them in taxes. It is getting more and more difficult for us all, professionals and consumers, to get together to produce research results in a way that district managers of the future are going to understand. This was underlined by Professor Maynard who said that as a health authority person, he needed evidence to show whether midwives or obstetricians were the best people to provide maternity care.

We want a health service which is acceptable to the consumer, which is reasonably achieved and is cost-effective. The way to do that is with midwifery care and GP care. The problem is that those who make up the iron triangle have been saying that hospital delivery is the way forward for the last 30 years.

Professor Ham I think Wendy Savage is highlighting very clearly why we need to change the NHS. There is a good case for reform rather than leaving things as they are, keeping the iron triangles in place. The changes do offer the opportunity for greater transparency, greater openness about priority setting, much of which has been hidden in the past. Health authorities are going to have to stand up in public and defend their decisions, which will not be popular. In that position, it seems to me there is a new market for information and evidence about what works and what does not and how much it costs, which has not existed before. The incentive is a different one and arguably is a stronger one and that is why I think the Oregon experience is so relevant to us because our health authorities will not be able to escape taking those kinds of priority decisions. They will need to support their decisions by the evidence which has always existed but which people have either ignored or not used, because in the past we ran a provider-dominated health service in which medical views have been much more important than any receiver views; setting up purchasers is a way of beginning to challenge that.

Purchasing is the name on an empty box; the crucial question is what you put into that box. What are you purchasing for? Who are you purchasing for? There is an opportunity but no guarantee it will happen, to purchase far more cost-effective services, far more consumer-oriented services. Where are the battalions supporting the consumer groups; there are not any at the moment, but creating this clearer separation between health authorities and providers begins to open up an avenue for consumer groups to look to health authorities to use their purchasing power, to move services away from the iron triangles and to come up with some different kind of configuration.

Gavin Young (General Practitioner, Penrith) Professor Dingwall's suggestion that professionals know best and could end up prosecuting the mother for not caring for her baby during pregnancy and labour, seems to be the old adage of 'something's gone wrong, blame the patient'. For several reasons this is perturbing. We just do not have enough evidence to know when it is her fault. What, for instance, would have happened if this policy had been operational in the 1970s if a mother at 42 weeks had rejected the idea of induction of labour and her baby had died or been born brain-damaged? At that time, for then good reasons, we felt induction was necessary and she might well have been prosecuted using the evidence available at the time. In fact both these things, the policy of induction for post-maturity and our knowledge now that the vast majority of cerebral palsy has nothing to do with intrapartum events, makes a nonsense of that. What about a woman who smokes? Are we going to turn round and prosecute her rather than prosecute the Government for their feeble action on the advertising of tobacco. What about a woman who has an abortion? At what point is she allowed to have an abortion yet suddenly not allowed to decide what happens in late pregnancy?

Professor Dingwall I want to state that nowhere in my paper did I make any reference to the notion of prosecuting women. Indeed the whole basis of my thesis was to query what it would take to protect the children's interests without creating some sort of obstetric tyranny. It is important that we should effect the things that we can effect in this area, but that we should not bypass the changes we can make using campaigns of public education based on professional assessments of risk. We should not forget to inform the public about the dangers of smoking and alcohol, while we go in search of some Utopian reconstruction of the social order so that we just wave a magic wand, tobacco advertizing will disappear and people will just give up smoking overnight.

A note of caution on the nature of the information dysymmetrics in this area. The imbalance of information between professionals and patients is such that we should not simply assume that we ought to give consumers all they want or just tell them what they want to hear. A gross example was on television recently concerning the consumer demand in this country for hard-core pornography. Television journalists were interviewing punters wandering around Soho streets grumbling about how tame the movies were. A couple of very articulate women from the film centres were saying, that although that may be the case, nevertheless they thought that this sort of material is a form of degradation of women that is socially unacceptable; even if there is a market for it, it should not necessarily be met. In a strange way the same applies to health care, and particularly in obstetric care. There are some things which are simply unacceptable, and I do not think we should be obliged to cater for every consumer demand.

In our assessment of the risk–benefit ratio to one or other parties, we must remember that in this case it is the mother who is in the position to articulate the demand and the child who is not, and so is disfavoured. To accede to demand of the one would be to compromise severely the interests of the other. There is an important balance to be struck here and I make no apology for articulating the problem in this striking way. I do not for a moment however believe that the way to deal with this is by locking up mothers in the American fashion.

Section 2
Professional and public participation in policy-making

5

An obstetrician's view of the maternity services in the 1990s

Richard Beard

Since World War II there have been a number of reports on the maternity services in the NHS. The first confidential enquiry into maternal mortality published in 1957[1] revealed that women were continuing to die from haemorrhage, sepsis, and lack of availability of operative facilities. Not surprisingly Sir John Peel in 1970[2] wrote in his report 'Domiciliary Midwifery and Maternity Bed Needs' as follows: 'We think that sufficient facilities should be provided to allow 100% hospital delivery. The greater safety of hospital confinement for mother and child justifies this objective'. The ready availability of blood for transfusion, medical and surgical expertise and facilities in hospital supported his conclusion. Yet the acceptance of his report meant that, almost overnight, having a baby, which for the great majority of women had been a domestic affair, was converted into a medical affair by transferring events to hospital. It seemed right at the time that those with normal pregnancies should forego the benefits of home delivery in order to ensure the safety of the many women whose lives were threatened by unpredictable obstetric emergencies.

The medicalization of pregnancy continued over the next two decades. In 1974 the Oppé report[3] recommended that neonatal intensive care should be available throughout the country. In practice this has meant that the prognosis for the 8–10% of babies born prematurely improved immeasurably but at the same time the argument for having a baby in hospital was further strengthened.

In 1980 a report on perinatal and neonatal mortality was published from the Social Services Select Committee of the House of Commons, chaired by Mrs Renée Short[4]. This was a comprehensive assessment of the maternity services and ended by making 150 recommendations designed to improve the effectiveness of the existing services. It was followed by a report 'Maternity Care in Action'[5] from the DHSS Maternity Services Advisory Committee, 'designed to help health authorities to evaluate the services they provide, answer public criticism and assess the priority that should be accorded to remedying deficiencies. It should also enable them to check whether their resource is being used as effectively as possible'. In 1982 a recommendation from the Royal College of Obstetricians and Gynaecologists[6] (RCOG) 'to accommodate the wishes of pregnant women within the confines of safety for mother and child', underlined the difficult balance between ensuring that pregnancy was a good experience for the mother yet safeguarding clinical practice. The importance of a caring approach was emphasized in a report from a RCOG working party, 'The Management of Perinatal Deaths'[7]. Most recently the reorganization of the NHS embodied in the Government's White Paper has further emphasized the need for critical assessment of practice based on outcome by all professionals within the maternity services.

ISSUES LIKELY TO INFLUENCE THE MATERNITY SERVICES IN THE 1990s

These are summarized in Figure 1.

Safety

The safety of the maternity services in Britain is revealed by the progressive decline in perinatal mortality between 1975 and 1990 from 19.3 to 8.3 babies per 1000 births. Maternal mortality has shown an equally sharp fall between 1973 and 1975 and 1985 and 1987 from 18.2 to 7.6 women per 100 000 births.

Safety for mothers and babies remains the major issue for obstetricians in planning the maternity services for the 1990s. The significant improvements in maternal and perinatal mortality which occurred from 1940 onwards are generally ascribed to the introduction of antibiotics, readily available blood for transfusion, and safer anaesthesia. These are all obtainable in hospital and there is little doubt that a return to delivery outside hospital would seriously endanger the lives of those women who continue to have life-threatening complications of pregnancy. This is an issue that is well understood by the public who accept the limitations of hospital care as a family event in return for the greater sense of

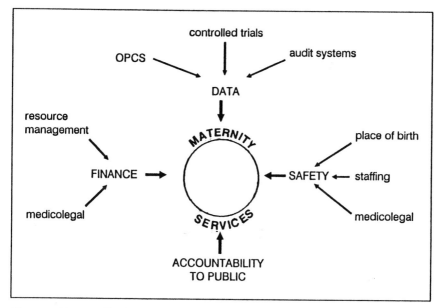

Figure 1 Issues affecting the development of the maternity services in the 1990s

security that accompanies delivery of a baby in hospital. Nevertheless, while the search for improved safety may be an objective of those who work in the maternity services, women also have a right to make an informed choice about the care they receive. It would be wrong to deny women, who do not accept the arguments for hospital delivery, the opportunity of having a home delivery that is as safe as possible. This means that it is essential for the hospital services to maintain a close link with those undertaking home delivery and to provide emergency cover as far as is possible.

The provision and quality of care are major factors in ensuring the safety of mother and baby. The current system whereby midwives, obstetricians, and paediatricians act as a team underlies this approach in Britain. The effectiveness of this system is dependent on many factors such as adequate staffing, availability of expertise, and harmonious working of the team. Both midwives and doctors are independent practitioners in their own right yet this should not prevent them working together for the benefit of mother and baby. Each have different roles with midwives providing the bulk of care to women with uncomplicated pregnancies, transferring responsibility to the obstetrician if complications develop. With the greater safety for mother and baby that has come with modern maternity care, the role of midwives needs to be expanded. Their potential as practitioners needs to be developed by the use of new technologies such as ultrasound, Doppler flow measurement, and greater involvement in the care of high-risk groups with conditions such as preterm labour, diabetes, and pregnancy-induced hypertension.

Education is an integral part of safe practice. The current system that exists in most maternity units whereby new medical staff learn by example from their seniors, is no longer adequate as the sole means of improving clinical competence. The increasing complexity of care and the heavy service load obstetricians bear does not provide time for more experienced clinicians to pass on their skills. The same is also true for midwives, particularly with the arrival of new technologies. An example of this is fetal monitoring. Midwives are expected to call for medical aid when a case is no longer normal. Unless they have received detailed instruction in fetal monitoring they cannot be expected to recognize when a fetal heart trace is abnormal. In the future, in-service education of medical and midwifery staff must become routine on all maternity units.

Accountability to the public

The maternity services provide care, by and large, for healthy young women. It is no longer acceptable to provide that care without the informed agreement of pregnant women and their partners. This can only be done by educating women before and during pregnancy so that they can take part in a realistic discussion about their care with those providing that care. Much has been achieved towards this end in recent years with the free distribution of the Health Education Authority's 'Pregnancy Book' and the widespread use of parentcraft classes as a part of antenatal care. However, with the advent of new technology, such as prenatal diagnosis, and neonatal intensive care, more and more issues of increasing complexity are presenting which take longer to explain to women. Time must be given in the maternity services for counselling which should have equal priority alongside the new developments of technology. Attitudes must also change amongst professionals to ensure that complexity of care is not used as an excuse to impose management without achieving some understanding by the woman of the issues involved.

Audit of practice

Recent changes in the NHS have laid justifiable emphasis on the importance of audit. The maternity services have always recognized this need, and audit in the form of a regular review of cases, perinatal mortality meetings and an annual report for maternity units, are a part of the range of activity which has been taking place for many years. Nevertheless, one has to question whether, in the past, effective use has been made of data derived from audit. Undoubtedly case conferences, the individual cases described in the confidential enquiries into maternal mortality and the many perinatal mortality surveys in recent years have, in a subconscious manner, contributed to improvements in clinical care. However, the outcome of pregnancy is so much safer than it used to be that any change in clinical practice such as a rise in Caesarean section rate has to be justified. It may be done in the name of greater safety, but such a change still has to be demonstrated as achieving this end. In the future a part of audit will be a comparison between maternity units of clinical and cost-effective outcome indicators. Clearly such an exercise must not become too rigorous because of a potentially dangerous loss of clinical freedom to respond to the needs of the individual case. Nevertheless, the development of large computerized databases makes such comparisons inevitable and the challenge for the 1990s is to make effective use of such data.

The other form of audit, on which increasing reliance will be placed to test the efficiency of clinical practice and procedures, is the randomized, controlled trial. Not all practices are amenable to this kind of testing. An example of this is the recent trial of method of delivery for preterm babies presenting by the breech, supported by Birthright. The clinicians did not feel that they were able, on ethical grounds, to randomize women to vaginal delivery or Caesarean section so that in the event sufficient cases could not be collected. It may be that in the future the large databases can be used to answer such difficult issues.

Medicolegal constraints

In a recent lecture at the Royal College of Midwives Sir Donald Acheson, the Chief Medical Officer, made some important points[8]. His figures showed a sharp increase in the cases involving brain-damaged infants that have come to the courts in recent years. Between 1983 and 1989 the number of such cases has risen from 50 a year to 157. He estimated that if this trend continues, it is probable that it would rise incrementally with a figure of at least 200 for 1990.

The significance of these trends is underlined by a survey amongst all consultant obstetricians and gynaecologists in Britain carried out by the Royal College of Obstetricians and Gynaecologists. It transpires that 85% have been sued at least once and that more than 60% have been sued more than once. These figures are worrying for a number of reasons. Of immediate concern to us is the damaging effect that such a climate of litigation has on the way obstetrics is practised and on the relationship between obstetricians and their patients.

In the USA the high level of settlements and the consequent rise in premiums for medical insurance, has resulted in a rapid decline in doctors prepared to practise obstetrics outside hospital. Patients are encouraged to sue by their lawyers and this has inevitably led to the emergence of a form of defensive medicine which is not good for the patient or the doctor.

In Britain, with a National Health Service, the implications of high settlements are somewhat different from the USA. Here, health authorities indemnify the hospital practitioner and all costs have to be paid out of revenue received for patient care. Recent figures from the Medical Protection Society show, for instance, that obstetricians and gynaecologists were involved in almost 30% of cases for which damages were paid. When one realizes that of the 60 000 practitioners in Britain only 2.5% of medical practitioners are engaged in obstetrics, this further underlines the crisis we have in the specialty.

The high level of awards is also worrying because of the drain on revenue for the hospital services. Last year it was estimated that at least 200 cases claiming obstetric negligence will reach the courts and more will be settled out of court. In 1989, the average settlement of such a case was £700 000 and many more cases were settled out of court. This means that in any given year many health authorities, even if they have only one settlement for a case brought against one of their obstetricians, will face a bill that will seriously interfere with the quality of care they provide.

What is the cause of all this litigation? One could reasonably claim that there is 'no smoke without fire'. Is there, for example, any evidence that a change in the clinical practice of obstetricians could account for this increase in litigation? This seems unlikely because both the perinatal mortality and maternal mortality rates have never been lower. Alternatively, have the public started to sue when in the past they did not? This explanation seems more credible because many long-standing cases are now being brought to court. Recent figures on cerebral palsy show that 28% of cases involve children delivered more than 5 years ago, some as long as 20 years ago. It is also relevant to ask why the public, who in the past have generally been so supportive of the medical profession, have suddenly started to attack obstetricians through the courts? The answer is not simple, and here the experience in the USA is useful. It would seem from that experience that, while the majority of litigants have a grievance that they wish to see put right, high awards against the medical profession do encourage lawyers and patients to sue.

The solution to the problem is far from clear, but a number of things can be done to improve matters. A recent article in the *British Medical Journal* by Ennis and Vincent[9] on behalf of the Medical Protection Society, revealed that in 64 cases of perinatal or maternal death, and of neurological damage to the baby, that came to litigation between 1982 and 1986, there were three major issues of concern: inadequate supervision of practice by senior staff; mismanagement of forceps delivery, and inadequate fetal monitoring. Looked at broadly, these cases reveal that all maternity units need to review the way in which obstetric care is provided. Does the system of medical and midwifery cover of a nerve centre like the labour ward ensure that experienced staff are available at all times 24 hours a day? Are new staff adequately trained in and familiarized with the various aspects of routine care such as fetal monitoring and operative delivery? These issues generate further questions about staffing levels particularly involving midwives who provide the bulk of labour ward care. There is also the problem of reduced availability of senior staff working on more than one site.

These are a few of the long-standing problems in the provision of maternity care that can be addressed by the profession. How we can avoid going further down the path of maternity care in the USA is at present not clear.

Resource management

The new NHS offers exciting challenges and some daunting restrictions. Obstetricians, often aided by their midwifery colleagues as business managers, have become clinical directors with control over the maternity budget. The potential for improvement lies in the possibility of better organization of services. Midwifery and medical staff can be deployed more effectively and money can be taken from activities of low priority to fund new developments. The danger of resource management is that no one as yet knows what is an appropriate budget for a service, and in many cases, with the rapidly developing maternity services, it is likely to be too low. The view of the profession is divided on the value of these developments, yet it cannot be denied that for the first time obstetricians and midwives have the opportunity to influence resources to the benefit of mothers and babies in a way that has not been possible before. It is an opportunity of the 1990s that is not to be missed.

REFERENCES

1. Ministry of Health. (1957). Report on Confidential Enquiries into Maternal Deaths in England and Wales 1952–54. *Reports on Public Health and Medical Subjects, No. 97.* (London: HMSO)
2. Department of Health and Social Security and the Welsh Office. Central Health Services Council. Standing Maternity and Midwifery Advisory Committee (Chairman Sir John Peel). (1970). *Domiciliary Midwifery and Maternity Bed Needs. Report of the sub-committee*
3. Department of Health and Social Security (Chairman, Professor T.E. Oppé). (1974). *Report of the Working Party on the Prevention of Early Neonatal Mortality and Morbidity.* (London: DHSS)
4. House of Commons, Social Services Committee (Chairman, Mrs Renée Short). (1980). *Second Report: Perinatal and Neonatal Mortality, Vol 1.* (London: HMSO)
5. Maternity Services Advisory Committee (Chairman, Mrs Alison Munro). (1984). *Second Report: Maternity Care in Action. Part 2: Care During Childbirth (Intrapartum Care).* (London: HMSO)
6. Royal College of Obstetricians and Gynaecologists. (1982). *Report of the RCOG Working Party on Antenatal and Intrapartum Care.* (Chairman, Professor M.C. MacNaughton). (London: RCOG)
7. Royal College of Obstetricians and Gynaecologists. (1985). *Report of the Working Party on the Management of Perinatal Deaths.* (Chairman, Mr R.D. Atlay). (London: RCOG)
8. Acheson, D. (1990). William Power Memorial Lecture. Presented to the Royal College of Midwives, December 1990
9. Ennis, M. and Vincent, C. (1990). Obstetric accidents – a review of 64 cases. *Br. Med. J.,* **300,** 1365–7

6

The midwife's contribution

Margaret Brain

Among the professionals involved in the maternity services, midwives are unique in several ways. This determines their essential role and contribution in policy-making.

THE MIDWIFE'S PLACE

The uniqueness of the midwife's role stems from the fact that she has chosen to prepare herself to be 'with woman', the literal meaning of the word 'midwife'. Through her education and training she accepts responsibility for caring for women in their reproductive lives and for promoting health for them and their babies. Her training is geared towards supporting and assisting healthy women who are experiencing a normal life event. This is in no way to denigrate the role of doctors whose training in the main is concerned with pathology and disease. I respect their scientific and technical skills. One only has to see the joy on the face of a high-risk woman safely delivered of a much wanted child to appreciate the full value of the medical role.

Midwives are almost an exclusively female profession caring for an exclusively female group of service users. They therefore have a legitimate interest in a range of women's issues which go far beyond the maternity services. They have views on women's reproductive health, on social welfare, child care provision, housing, employment rights and public health matters. Midwives are concerned with the impact of all such Government policies on women's social, political and economic lives, for they impinge on the midwife's everyday work and may lead to specific interventions. It is now well recognized that the outcome of pregnancy is dependent not only on the organization and quality of the maternity services but also on the social policies of Government which affect public health.

How do midwives influence these wider policy decisions? The Royal College of Midwives (RCM) has a permanent seat on the Women's National Commission. This was set up some 21 years ago 'to ensure by all possible means that the informed opinions of women are given their due weight in the deliberations of Government'. Participation in the work of the Commission is one way in which the views of midwives on all legislative matters are made known.

Midwives are the only professionals who work in consultant maternity units, in general practitioner (GP) units, in health centres, GP surgeries and in the home. In fact the midwife will be 'with woman' wherever the woman is during her pregnancy, labour and afterwards. They are therefore concerned with the total maternity service – primary, secondary and tertiary.

THE MATERNITY SERVICES

When considering pregnancy care for the 1990s we are looking at a wide range of services and options. They are now so extensive that all the professionals involved must target their energies so that optimum use may be made of their skills. In planning services we must remember that women's cultural, social and medical needs are so diverse that we cannot reduce options without seriously affecting the outcome of birth and/or the level of consumer satisfaction. As women have fewer children their expectations rise. They want every prospect of a healthy baby but they also want their pregnancy and childbirth to be recognized as a normal life event which completes their womanhood and builds their family. Women from ethnic minorities, women with marginal fertility, women with pregnancies which a few years ago would have appeared impossible to sustain – all require services tailored to their needs.

Modern women are also workers. There is therefore a real cost to them and to their employers if their pregnancy care is inadequate. They need a high health status throughout pregnancy and throughout the postnatal period, and they need care which is convenient and appropriate to them as individuals.

A recent report, 'Maternity Rights: the Experience of Women and Employers'[1] indicated that today twice as many women go back to work after having a baby as did 10 years ago. Many more women are working full-time. It is crucial that the care we professionals plan and offer is care which fits their needs. We cannot, and indeed must not, expect them to alter their lives to fit into our systems of care if we believe in the value of the care we give. For the Royal College of Midwives' Annual Conference this year, our branches have selected a motion urging the Government to support the provisions of the draft EEC directive on the protection of pregnant women at work and to make changes to ratify its provisions.

The professionals involved in the maternity services need to recognize each others' complementary but distinct roles and responsibilities. Many reports have commented on the duplication of services and the failure to make full use of resources. The managers of the new NHS with its market orientation will be alert to service specifications which appear to duplicate care. We cannot simply say we need more doctors, we need more midwives. Maybe we do, but the demographic and economic factors suggest we will not get them, and our only choice is to get together to establish and agree appropriate methods of working.

Throughout the world maternity care is receiving special attention. The International Safe Motherhood Initiative launched in 1987 called on all countries of the world to take action to reduce maternal mortality and make motherhood safe for all. There is a consensus among international funding agencies that to promote safe motherhood requires a worker who is 'with woman' in her own community and who provides care throughout pregnancy and childbirth. In fact what is required is a worker modelled on the British midwife. In the developed world too there has been a new understanding of the contribution the midwife can make. For example until recently maternity care in Canada was physician-centred with birth taking place in hospital. Provincial governments are now looking at midwifery care as an alternative to physician care in low-risk pregnancies and at birthing centres as an alternative to hospital labour wards.

So it is generally agreed that Midwifery is a Good Thing!

You will recall that in the early 1980s, the Maternity Services Advisory Committee (MSAC) emphasized the need to make effective use of midwives' skills. The recommendations in its reports[2-4] remain Government policy today. More recently, in 'Working for Patients'[5], the Government reiterated in the section on managing resources the need to make full use of the midwives as recommended in the MSAC reports.

POLICY-MAKING SYSTEMS

In considering the midwives' contribution to policy-making it is not only necessary for us to know where the policy decisions are made but also how the system works.

Service provision is about planning and practice. Choices will always have to be made; policies will be concerned with the type of service. Is it to be medically oriented or midwifery oriented? Is it to be hospital-centred or community-centred? Or is it to be woman-centred? Will it concentrate on large centralized delivery suites or small community units? These questions are not simply technical ones concerned with perceived good outcomes of a particular type of service; they are political questions. Choices have to be made and a balance found between professional expectations and government philosophies.

What do we need to do to influence policy decisions to ensure that each and every woman receives appropriate care? Policy decisions are made at Government level, in Regional and District Health Authorities and in individual hospitals and GP surgeries. Never before, or so it seems, has there been so much change in the Health Service. Fundamental changes are also taking place in Government itself. Such times of change however bring a climate of opportunity.

Under the Next Steps programme large parts of government machinery are being hived off into executive agencies with the aim of delivering better services more efficiently. Ultimately it is hoped that three-quarters of the Civil Service will switch to agency status leaving just a small core overseeing policy. This small Civil Service will no longer be able to develop and generate all policies. Gone will be the days when large numbers of Departmental policies are issued requiring consistency in implementation throughout the country. In this new era they will have to 'buy in' certain policies and the professional organizations must be alert to this opportunity.

THE MIDWIVES' CONTRIBUTION

As midwives we are ready. The RCM in 1987 produced a policy statement for the maternity services entitled *Towards a Healthy Nation*. It provides the framework for the pattern of care which we believe is needed in the 1990s if women are to be full and equal partners in a service which is both flexible and readily available. We have recently reviewed this publication[6]. Having established a good framework we are now ready to promote the type of service we believe in and can quickly respond to any call for statements or for evidence to Government committees. It is very important that such advice is consistent with earlier advice. One should lead on from the other, fitting into a framework in a logical and consistent manner.

Could midwives practise midwifery better? I think most would agree we could. One of the most controlling factors for midwives is the design of the service in which they have to operate. Health authority policies can be restricting as well as enabling. At national level this is influenced by legislation. Midwives practise under primary legislation[7] which exists independently from any legislation governing the NHS. However, how they are able to practise depends to a great extent on the local arrangements for the maternity services.

At regional and district health authority levels there must be a midwife of sufficient standing and seniority to speak up for midwives and to ensure that local services facilitate midwives' fulfilling their proper role. In the new NHS the purchasers and the providers have been organizationally and sometimes geographically separated. Central to the successful implementation of the White Paper[5] is the opportunity to specify the quality of the service being bought and sold, or purchased and provided. We welcomed the appointment of a midwife on the newly formed National Clinical Standards Advisory Committee.

The RCM has and will continue to contribute to discussions on the formulation of contracts. Duncan Nichol, the NHS Chief Executive, made it quite clear in his letter to all general managers last December[8] that the views and broad support of staff regarding the contracts was necessary. He repeated earlier advice that: 'The active involvement of clinicians and others will be required in drawing up the service and quality specification elements of contracts'.

THE DRAFT CONTRACTS

The RCM took part in advising Ministers and the Department on the various draft contracts, checking to see that they enable midwives to fulfil their role in the interests of the women for whom the service is being designed. Specifically we are looking for the service:

(1) To be provided close to the women's homes;

(2) To be integrated to allow women to receive continuity of care by practitioners they know; and

(3) To be one in which the midwife is enabled to utilize fully and appropriately all her skills to meet the needs to both low-risk and high-risk women.

FUTURE POLICIES

So what changes in policies for pregnancy care in the 1990s do midwives want?

Firstly, they want a service designed for women, not designed for Government, for health authorities or for the professions. They want one designed for the actual users of the service – the women. This is in line with the consumerism outlined in the White Paper[5]. High priority must be given to providing women with the care they want.

Secondly, the package of care must include a whole range of services. It must be remembered that all pregnant women do not need or want the same type of care. The low risk, the medically at risk and the socially at risk all require a different package of care with different inputs from all of the professionals concerned.

Thirdly, the service must include the option of a midwifery model of care. At the onset of pregnancy the woman must be able to decide to refer herself to a midwife or to a doctor. This does not imply that either GPs or midwives should provide care in isolation from each other. The midwife will refer to the GP for the provision of general health care needs and will refer directly to the consultant obstetrician if complications arise or specific advice is requested.

For this easy access to a midwife, midwifery clinics must be established where women congregate so that they are easily accessible. Those in certain branches of Boots and Mothercare are fulfilling a real need. This midwifery model will also include midwifery beds in all consultant and GP maternity units for use for an increased number of 'Domino' deliveries and for women who choose to have longer stays.

Parliamentarians from meetings with their constituents and from their extensive postbags are well aware of the continuing debate on the way women receive maternity care. It is no accident that the Health Committee which could have looked at any one of a number of important health issues has chosen as its first topic the maternity services. This is an important arena in which the conflicting issues surrounding the best way of providing maternity care can be fully aired. All will have the opportunity to present evidence. For the first time this Health Committee has appointed two midwife advisers among its professional advisers. Hopefully its report will help everybody concerned to move towards a consensus.

I hope the care we all provide over the next 10 years will be truly woman-centred and will meet her physical, social, emotional and educational needs.

REFERENCES

1. McRae, S. and Daniel, W.W. (1991). *Maternity Rights: The Experience of Women and Employers*. (London: Policy Studies Institute)

2. Maternity Services Advisory Committee. (1982). *Maternity Care in Action. Part 1: Antenatal care.* (London: HMSO)
3. Maternity Services Advisory Committee. (1984). *Maternity Care in Action. Part 2: Care during Childbirth (Intrapartum Care).* (London: HMSO)
4. Maternity Services Advisory Committee. (1985). *Maternity Care in Action. Part 3: Care of the Mother and Baby (Postnatal and Neonatal Care).* (London: HMSO)
5. Department of Health and Social Security. (1989). *Working for Patients.* (London: HMSO)
6. Royal College of Midwives. (1990). *Towards a Healthy Nation.* (London: RCM)
7. *Nurses, Midwives and Health Visitors Act.* (1979). (London: HMSO)
8. Chief Executive, NHS. (1990). Management Executive Letter to General Managers, EL (90) 221

7
General practitioner participation in policy-making

Peter Kielty

This contribution is devoted to medical support for confinement managed in the community, i.e. in small GP maternity units and the home. Today, antenatal and postnatal care are fully developed, non-controversial parts of general practice and need no more than our continued support. On the other hand, decisions must be taken very soon about home and small unit confinement lest they disappear for ever.

THE PLACE OF THE GP

GPs are fairly accommodating people. Traditionally they serve the perceived needs of people in their communities, without too much concern for analysis and policy-making. In this country, at least, they are always there, part of the equation which must be considered by those involved in planning. General practice is an influence more than a participant.

To understand our present dilemma we need to be clear about what GPs are and how they themselves are influenced by policy changes. Firstly, they serve communities where they live, working at street level, caring for people they already know, before, during and after each episode of illness or pregnancy. This influence on them has never been quantified but I am sure that it matters.

Secondly, they are self-employed contractors, paid through fees and allowances which can be changed, both to reflect changing circumstances and to modify incentives to fit in with policy. Government frequently does this and, maternity care apart, has just made many radical changes to the GPs' contract.

Thirdly, GPs do many things besides provide maternity care. This forms only a small part of the average doctor's work and remuneration; not everybody is involved and nobody needs to be.

Historically, GPs are more subject to policy decisions of others than they are policy-makers themselves, but they are always there, and those who plan must always take account of their contribution. Sometimes they were useful. Before the Health Service started in 1948, they were useful to midwives who needed medical help; £3 for suturing a perineum or £2 for resuscitating a baby – such were the priorities. Available again in 1948, GPs solved the Government's problems with maternity care within the new Health Service, being happy to provide continuous care from booking to a postnatal examination for seven guineas. The antenatal checks were specified: half-a-guinea each or 52½p.

Yet again GPs were there following the Cranbrook report, welcoming coordination with obstetricians and the greater emphasis placed on antenatal care. The new GP fee structure devoted 60% of the maximum to antenatal care, rather than the 30% or so of the past, while retaining a confinement fee which was respectable enough at the time. Once again changes got results, GPs adapted, morale rose and perinatal mortality fell.

Sadly, that is about where influence, accommodation and incentive came to an end. Since that time we have failed to address the role of the GP properly and the arrangements for GPs have become frozen in time. The 1958 Perinatal Mortality Survey of the National Birthday Trust generated a whole series of events which, accompanied by the growing power of the Royal College of Obstetricians and Gynaecologists (RCOG), served to exclude GPs from intrapartum care in the community, progressively leaving community midwives with fewer doctors with the expertise to assist at the few confinements they manage to retain. Expertise withers without constant practice, and community deliveries have practically disappeared in many areas. Where they still exist they have, as part of our new consumerist health service, become a loss-leader.

It need not have happened. Proper training in the new techniques suitable for community use, a greater understanding and development of case selection and a proper adjustment to the fee for confinement relative to the increased responsibility were the changes we should have anticipated and they should have been worked on as they had in the past.

Instead we entered a new era of steady deterioration, crying out for change. The Government will not make changes without professional consensus for change and despite every effort, particularly in the last 10 years since the last conference (Pregnancy Care in the 1980s), and since the joint report of the RCOG and the Royal College of General Practitioners (RCGP) (1980), it has not been possible to reach agreement.

At the same time, GP trainees have been reared in their senior house officer training posts on a diet of abnormality and fear, sufficient to discourage them for life. New doctors today never were steeped in blood and liquor as students in the way that we older ones were, and they really do believe that all maternity care is abnormal. It may not be too long before the RCGP reaches the conclusion that maternity training for general practice, as it is currently organized in hospitals, is no longer appropriate, and states a preference for training by GP obstetricians and teaching midwives in the community. After all, these are the people who currently retrain new doctors in practice and get out of their heads most of the perspectives introduced by hospital programming.

Without this there will soon be no medical support in the community. Already we have seen obstetricians in West Berkshire finding their local GPs unable to facilitate home confinements when the unit was overbooked, so diminished was their expertise and confidence. In our new cash and carry Health Service this will happen everywhere just as soon as a moderate increase in birth rate occurs. A greater increase than that and we will all be in the headlines as part of a new national medical crisis. Decisions and changes must therefore be made quickly, and not just by professionals as we should all remember that the community will also wish to have a say in the ultimate decisions.

THE FUTURE OF GP OBSTETRICS

The Health Committee of the House of Commons, currently looking at provisions for normal pregnancy and confinement, will soon make recommendations. One can think of four possibilities.

(1) That a medical component in the community is no longer necessary? Leave it all to the midwives, the ambulance service and pray for an open road. Not all midwives would welcome that and not all mothers either.

(2) Is there a new role for consultant obstetricians, with personal availability to the community 24 hours a day? This is unlikely.

(3) Can we rely on the present obligation on ill-trained and unmotivated GPs to do their best, a situation which is already worse in some areas than conditions which existed before the Health Service began? It is unlikely that the Health Committee will wish to do this for it really means making no proposal at all about this matter.

(4) Perhaps the Committee will suggest that together with the Government, the medical profession should start sensible discussion with a view to recovering the situation through acceptable agreements on training, on standards and incentives.

Possibly we are already too late. In contrast with former times, GPs are no longer there to recover this activity. In the last 20 years they have moved on and today they are organized more in terms of leisure time than of commitment to intrapartum obstetrics in the community. Larger partnerships and commercial deputizing are greater influences than they were, and both are known impediments to any plans for revitalizing GP maternity care. Also GPs, struggling with the Department's new contract, have new priorities to consume their energies. They are no longer there to respond to polite requests and financial incentive.

What is more, the signs are not encouraging anyway. There was general agreement on a new joint report from the two colleges (RCOG and RCGP) which contains a number of sensible proposals. One proposal in particular would have replaced an outdated and inadequate criterion for admission to our obstetric list with a much more demanding module of community-based training for those doctors who have not been able to obtain a Senior House Officer (SHO) post; this has recently been turned down by the Council of the RCOG. There seems to be a problem with attitudes and it may be that for the first time GPs will not be influenced as they have been in the past, and today would not be willing to restart the discussions. There is a grave danger that this is the case.

Before such discussions can happen, attitudes must change lest those who hold them find their SHO numbers dwindling away and that they inherit the workload to add to their present difficulties. This is no way to proceed; surely we can restart the dialogue, improve the standards, change the training, remove the fear, and emerge with a united profession, with GPs no longer afraid of involvement in the community, and obstetricians free to concentrate on the real problems, uncluttered by a misplaced sense of responsibility to those who do not need their help.

8

Priorities in maternity health care: a paediatric view

Malcolm Levene

There are approximately 650 000 babies born in Britain every year and the vast majority of these are healthy and without abnormality. They will be routinely examined by either midwives or doctors, but otherwise require no professional attention in hospital. Those babies that do require paediatric attention include the 6% who are born prematurely as well as some full-term infants who have medical or surgical problems. About 10% of newborn babies require nursing on a special care baby unit, and approximately 2–3% of all births require neonatal intensive care. Development of skills and techniques has been associated with considerable improvement in the neonatal survival rates for premature infants. In the 20 years since 1965 the survival rate for babies born with a birth weight below 1000 g has increased from 16% to over 40% and the perinatal mortality rate for all liveborn and stillborn infants over the 10-year period 1976–86 has fallen from 18 to 10 per 1000 total births.

These improvements indicate that there has been an increase in standards nationally. In this time there has also been increased centralization of neonatal facilities within regional and sub-regional units. Paediatricians have been at the forefront of policy-making in order to encourage the development of a blueprint for neonatal services. The routes by which policy has been produced can be considered at a macro (national) and a micro (unit or health district) level.

National policy-making has occurred at Government level and at the instigation of professional groups. In the last 20 years a number of Government committees have been set up to report on neonatal services including:

(1) 1971, the Expert Group on Special Care for Babies. (The Sheldon Report);

(2) 1974, the Report of the Working Party on the Prevention of Early Neonatal Mortality and Morbidity (The Oppé Report);

(3) 1976, the Report of the Committee on Child Health Services (The Court Report);

(4) 1980, the House of Commons Social Services Select Committee (The Short Report); and,

(5) 1990, the Scottish Home and Health Department Report on Neonatal Care in Scotland.

In addition to these Reports, there have been a number of initiatives from paediatric professional bodies including:

(1) 1977, the Liaison Committee of the British Paediatric Association (BPA) and Royal College of Obstetricians and Gynaecologists (RCOG), 'Recommendations for the Improvement of Infant Care during the Perinatal Period in the UK';

(2) 1983, BPA and the British Association of Perinatal Medicine (BAPM), 'Categories of Babies Requiring Neonatal Care'; and,

(3) 1988, The Royal College of Physicians, 'Medical Care of the Newborn in England and Wales'.

Both Government and professional groups recommended a tiered system for delivering neonatal care. This included having paediatric facilities available in every hospital where babies were born. In district general hospitals, special care baby units should be set up to offer a level of care to small babies or those who were moderately sick. These babies often require careful observation by nursing and medical staff experienced in the care of the newborn unit. In addition each regional health authority should ensure that there are one or two regional neonatal intensive care units and three or four subregional units to give intensive care in the busier district general hospitals. Recommendations for staffing these units were also made. It has been generally agreed that progress in neonatal care is best made within this tiered structure.

The regional health authorities, responsible for organizing the care of 40000–60000 deliveries per year have acted with no great haste to implement these recommendations or to overview the development of neonatal care under their responsibility and in some regions neonatal services have evolved at a faster or slower rate. Unfortunately, despite agreed recommendations, the national blueprint has not emerged as a coherent policy.

At the micro level, the district health authorities (DHAs) have organized services in a piecemeal fashion. Larger DHAs have spent money on neonatal intensive care cots and the smaller ones have tended to send babies away for neonatal intensive care to large districts or the regionally funded neonatal intensive care units. In some regions the neonatal services in the various DHAs have developed or contracted depending on local factors, but not in a coordinated fashion.

Many of the smaller DHAs have found it impossible to stretch their facilities to provide a good service for newborn infants. Their dilemma is that the needs are greater than the provision. An example is the need for relatively experienced, paediatrically trained doctors immediately available for resuscitation wherever babies are born. In addition skilled paediatricians must be available in special care baby units for the emergencies that irregularly occur. In some districts, the maternity unit may be situated some way from the baby unit or even in another hospital.

The provision is inadequate in that the junior paediatric doctors on call for resuscitation are often GP trainees who are only responsible for paediatrics for 6 months and who never achieve the level of skills necessary to provide safe cover. In addition there are few middle grade doctors on paediatric cover. This means that the consultant paediatrician must be available for emergencies, and when there are only two or three per district, it is clear that a safe service cannot be guaranteed all of the time.

The picture is emerging that macro policies advise that there must be a regional blueprint for neonatal care, but because the RHAs have not acted in concert, the services emerging at the micro level leave large holes in the perceived safety net. In other words there is a clear imbalance between expectations and actualities, and between the national blueprints and fine detail.

THE FUTURE

Unfortunately, with the introduction of the NHS and Community Services Act in 1991, the RHA requirement to oversee neonatal services may have been further subverted. Individual hospitals may decide to become providers of neonatal intensive care by buying in equipment and possibly staff. This will further encourage piecemeal development of neonatal services and hinder regionally supervised expansion.

The future policy for neonatal care must consider national strategic planning, regional strategic planning, identified central funding for neonatal care, and manpower expansion for safe care in all DHAs. Paediatricians must strive to influence Government and their professional bodies to identify priorities in neonatal health care planning in the areas suggested above.

9

Participation in policy-making: the maternity service users

Mary Newburn

How can women have a say in the kind of maternity services offered to them? Put more formally, how can recipients of care or maternity service users participate effectively in policy-making? In order to participate, service users must be able to influence those who have the power to make decisions and be able to work with them. When the Maternity Services Advisory Committee recommended that multidisciplinary Maternity Services Liaison Committees (MSLCs) should be set up at District level, including 'users or representatives of users' and drawing on their experience[1-3], this seemed like an important opportunity.

Over the intervening years numerous National Childbirth Trust (NCT) members have succeeded in getting a place on an MSLC, some by way of membership of their local Community Health Council (CHC). The evidence presented here comes from 41 accounts sent in earlier this year from members on health committees; 32 were from current or recent members of an MSLC or similar body.

Before going into what NCT user representatives had to say, it is important to note the recommended terms of reference for MSLCs laid down in the Maternity Care in Action reports. Perhaps most significantly they said:

> 'While Maternity Service Liaison Committees have an important advisory role, it is the Health Authorities which have the responsibility for ensuring the provision of adequate maternity services'[2].

Or as Garcia[4] put it:

'MSLCs were set up to advise decision-makers at district health authority level. They do not have the power to allocate resources or implement policy changes.'

Furthermore it was laid down that the committees might:

'... wish to meet in two forms: as a professional group when clinical and confidential matters or individual cases are to be discussed and with a wider membership including lay people ... for all other purposes'[2].

These two characteristics, an absence of power and a two-tier structure, have undoubtedly limited the opportunities of services users to participate in policy-making in many areas. One respondent wrote:

'... the real problem was with the lack of responsibility and budget rather than the unwillingness of people to talk and discuss issues.'

Another commented:

'All policy matters are decided at District Obstetric Liaison Committee to which lay members are not admitted.'

And a third:

'This committee had one meeting in January 1990, which was not minuted ... and did not meet again during the whole year as a full committee. (I think there were 'core group' meetings to which I am not normally invited).'

In addition, the financial straits in which health authorities and boards have found themselves have been a further negative pressure on the effectiveness of MSLCs:

'... we liaised with medical professionals and drew up a consensus agreement on the way forward for obstetrics in our area. However, the Health Board have yet to take this issue in hand and just ignore the whole maternity question. As you probably know this Health Board has overspent to the tune of £2.2 million.'

In summary, it would seem that MSLCs were intended to be an important means by which user representatives could discuss service provision with clinicians and managers and expect action to be taken as a result of the committee's recommendations. However, the guidelines for MSLCs meant that user representatives might be excluded from key meetings and the advice of the committee could be ignored by health authorities.

Bearing these limitations in mind, what have been the achievements and further obstacles experienced by users aiming to affect local maternity policies?

NCT MEMBERS' EXPERIENCES

At the positive end of the spectrum, it seems that MSLCs can genuinely be a local multidisciplinary forum for determining key aspects of maternity policy, with an increasing role for the user. One respondent said that on occasion, agenda items had been held over because users had sent apologies for absence; another listed among projects she had been involved in:

'looking at facilities for home deliveries, provision of birthing pools and stools, waiting times in antenatal clinics and provision of facilities for mothers and children waiting.'

Yet another, writing about the agreed arrangements following NHS review changes said that:

'The MSLC covering the whole DHA will meet four times a year with subcommittees ... meeting every six weeks at the two units to implement recommendations ... (and) users will ... be more strongly represented.'

She went on:

'I am beginning to feel more confident about pushing for more action in the MSLC and am hoping that with a more vigorous new chairperson and more user representation we will be more effective.'

The role on the MSLC of the chairperson was also referred to in the original Maternity Services Advisory Committee guidelines. The reports advised that MSLCs should be:

'properly led by a person of standing who is also an enthusiast for improvements'[1].

and added that the person should also have 'the time to make (the committee) work effectively'[2].

At the other end of the spectrum, where experiences were less positive, members reported a lack of enthusiasm among health professionals, and frequently mentioned a lack of commitment by the chairperson. The following quotes illustrate a range of experiences:

'The MSLC used to meet monthly but meetings were often cancelled due to lack of business! This I find very frustrating. Last September it was decided to meet three times a year ... The January meeting was cancelled so the next meeting will be May.'

'Sadly (our) MSLC is not a very productive body. ... Occasionally, views of the group are fed to the District Health Authority. ... Traditionally the chairman has been appointed from the DHA. They have declined to replace the outgoing chairman which I feel denotes a lack of importance.'

'The major obstacle, I feel, is the chairman as he sets the scene and tone of the meeting and tends to be quite dismissive of everyone's comments.'

'I have always felt the meetings to be totally unsatisfactory ... as it meets at lunchtime with members coming late, leaving early or answering bleeps during business, and to my mind the proceedings, such as they are, are not properly minuted.' (Perinatal Services Committee member).

'Meetings are usually more of a forum for male doctors to have their say with management over topical issues.'

These comments suggest that in many areas MSLCs are not taken seriously as policy advisory bodies and that the people chairing the committees would benefit from training.

On a brighter note, one MSLC member reported having had a significant effect within the committee. Though she had experienced obstetricians as 'rather patronising' at times, she said:

'I can speak openly, perhaps more so than other members who have to maintain working relations. For instance, when voting in a new chairman a few years ago the outgoing chairman, a consultant, said 'we usually alternate consultant and GP' to which I was able to butt in that I felt anybody could be chairman ... the midwifery manager was voted in as vice-chairman, and has since become chairman.'

In addition to infrequency of meetings, poor chairing, and difficulties in achieving right of access to policy meetings, members also reported meetings being held at inconvenient times, dates being altered at short notice and no provision for the payment of expenses for child care. Furthermore, despite the recommendation that the committee be 'assured of the support it needs to makes its work effective'[1], many are not well serviced. Hence user members must rely on their own resources and the local CHC for policy updates and other information. Yet, if user representatives are to work effectively they need to know the current issues and be in touch with research developments. Without structured support and without specific education or training for this work, the lone consumer on a committee can come unstuck. Some reported feeling very isolated and undermined. Alternatively a token parent with no relevant background knowledge beyond her own experience is likely to be ineffective.

Double standards often operate, under which a service user must be able to substantiate what she is talking about in order to be taken notice of, whereas others simply expect their opinions to carry sufficient weight. One woman wrote of her first MSLC meeting, when the topics on the agenda – home birth and water birth – attracted an unusually large turnout, including three GPs:

'It was these GPs who really flabbergasted me with their unsubstantiated attack on home births. They were totally against the option being available; one saying that he always managed to think up some reason over nine months as to why a woman should have to have a hospital confinement. ... He said women showed him statistics supporting home birth and that these statistics were flawed because (a) they inevitably came from Holland, and (b) the births were always low risk and therefore did not represent the true risk of mortality and morbidity. ... I did venture to suggest that there was British evidence suggesting that home births were safe and that home birth was primarily for the low-risk pregnancy. I received a withering look. Water birth was totally dismissed.'

Another woman wrote:

'As a consumer and CHC rep. I feel one has to work very hard to be taken seriously and get one's views heard. One of the consultants wrote a letter to me as an NCT member which implied the NCT was (subversively) pushing women into requests for delivery on all fours. We wrote a letter back stressing NCT's aims to enable informed choice, and quoting various articles about delivery positions and research indicating outcomes. Since then the particular consultant has treated me with more respect.'

User representatives are often in a minority on a committee of health professionals and managers, and even those clinicians who support the same issues are sometimes unwilling to speak out. The previous respondent went on to say:

'The midwives were enthusiastic about home birth but did not defend it at the meeting. I learned afterwards this was due to hospital politics. Indeed I was castigated (by them) for not having spoken up more.'

In a similar vein, another woman wrote:

'Originally the meetings were appalling. They were very much dominated by a couple of old-school consultants of the hellfire and brimstone variety. One of them literally slept through each meeting, only waking when someone said something he disagreed with. (People tended not to.) I well remember presenting the NCT Patients Charter to the Committee. I was demolished; torn apart and thrown on the scrap heap in about 10 seconds. (However, almost every member of the committee expressed their support for the charter in private.)'

Internal politics were often mentioned as a factor which blocked policy developments, typically between clinicians and managers or between doctors and midwives. As one example:

'I feel that own interests, particularly in the case of consultants, have affected the way they view care. ... I have supported the midwives' wish to take more responsibility for care, a view shared by the hospital manager (it is cheaper), but it has largely been met with resistance by the consultants and GPs.'

The picture presented here might lead one to question whether government thinking has changed since the reports of the Maternity Services Advisory Committee were published. However the National Audit Office report on Maternity Services[5], indicates that the Department of Health annual guidelines for 1989–90 urged improvements in maternity care, including 'more attention to users' views and wishes.'

The National Audit Office undertook to analyse the extent of compliance with the guidance laid down in the three Maternity Services Advisory Committee reports. From the surveys returned by districts, they found 93% claimed to have established an MSLC, but that frequency of meetings was reported to range from once to 24 times a year[5]. Unfortunately, this degree of inconsistency was not taken up by the Public Accounts Committee[6] when questioning Duncan Nichol, NHS chief executive, on the shortcomings detailed by the report.

NHS REVIEW

A discussion of this kind would not be complete without reference to the NHS review. Many respondents referred to the effect of NHS reorganization. Some felt the changes were going to yield an opportunity for increased user input but others were very concerned about accountability, choice and standards. In some areas MSLCs had been disbanded altogether, as the following two reports stated:

'I was involved in the setting up of a maternity satisfaction survey but in October they disbanded the MSLC.'

'Our MSLC was disbanded last year as the Government's White Paper was implemented.'

Though little or no reference was made to MSLCs in the NHS White Paper, the Department of Health has stated that the advisory role of MSLCs is to continue as before (P. Jenkins, Department of Health, 12th March 1991, personal communication).

Reports from those areas where MSLCs are continuing, revealed considerable variation in the arrangements being implemented. In some it seems the MSLC is to be a body of the purchaser, in others of the provider and sometimes of both. For example:

'Since the purchaser/provider split there's been a subtle change of alliances on the MSLC: providers seeing they have more in common with the CHC and consumers, and seeking CHC support to lobby purchasers.'

Another member wrote:

'Now things may be looking up. The Health Authority has decided that the MSLC will be a purchaser committee, monitoring services for the area. Added to this the consultants on the new committee include the husband of one of our antenatal teachers and another very go-ahead young man. Also our new Manager of Obstetrics and Gynaecology is a midwife and not averse to change. Their first request at the first meeting was for an NCT rep., as well as a CHC one. We left the meeting having decided to review the entire service – with investigations by the CHC/NCT as a major input into services.'

However, another letter made more depressing reading:

'Now with the purchaser/provider and directorate system, DHAs do not exist with the same consumer representation. Self-governing trusts will produce almost total autonomy. Our hospital does not need to make any concessions to clients because it is over-subscribed. The other hospital is 'open' because they are fighting for survival. It feels like a case of 'big boys' rule. The CHC is powerless because everything is based on money.'

It seems therefore that there are new problems afoot for service users. Though the government has said services should be responsive to patients' needs they have not built in mechanisms to ensure that the views of service users will be known, still less acted upon. These deficiencies have been documented elsewhere; however, it bears repeating that the user of maternity services is not the purchaser. The concerns of district health authorities and GP budget holders are not going to be the same concerns as those of women having babies.

District health authorities are now made up of fewer democratically elected people and more who have no specific interest in health care. Yet, community health councils have actually lost the right to be heard at health authority meetings and the right to visit outside their own area.

RECOMMENDATIONS

What can be done during the 1990s to ensure service users can participate in policy-making?

(1) The government must be lobbied to support, rather than undermine, CHCs; to clarify the role of MSLC, and to put pressure on health authorities; or, better still, to make it a requirement of health authorities that they institute an active MSLC in which service users are integral. The Health Select Committee is currently inquiring into maternity services and I trust it will make recommendations on this matter a priority.

(2) The publication of maternity statistics within regions will put local services in perspective and lend weight to arguments for improvements. The outcome of clinical audit should also be more widely available.

(3) Training should be developed and funded for service user representatives, and more women with a special interest in maternity issues should put themselves forward to serve on district health authorities and the advisory boards of hospital trusts. One of our members who has done so said:

'The only way to influence is to get people onto the policy-making bodies, but also to provide the training they are going to need to fight the business people who occupy the majority of the non-executive positions. We need to be able to fight as equals, the day of the consumer point of view put forward by volunteers has gone.'

(4)   Women and their families should be encouraged to write letters of praise and complaint to managers, midwives, consultants, CHCs, MPs, to organizations like the NCT, Maternity Alliance and AIMS, and to newspapers. Women's consciousness has been raised. They are less prepared just to accept the status quo these days.

(5)   Local user-groups may feel they are fighting a losing battle, but this has been the position in the past and positive change has been achieved. If direct consultation and participation in policy-making is not possible, achievable targets can be set. It may be possible to influence policy indirectly. An alliance of user organizations can set its own agenda and invite managers and clinicians to meet with it. In one area where this was done complaints received by the CHC were tabled for discussion each time and relationships with health professionals have improved.

In particular, contact with local midwives leading to regular meetings can be useful. Groups can also lobby for the government's standardized survey of women's experience of maternity care to be used in their area[7].

Though in many areas the gap between the perspective of service users and the stance of obstetricians seems a huge gulf, members wrote of the way in which the differences between midwives and childbearing women have been successfully overcome. On this subject, one said:

> 'Eight years ago we had the same problem with the midwives but now we can talk with them very openly and consider ourselves working towards common goals. So, it is worth persevering.'

This kind of achievement is the result of the patient, committed way in which service users have set about building open and constructive lines of communication. But it is also due in no small part to the way midwives have accepted the principle that women have a right to discuss services as equals, and their willingness in practice to make changes to accommodate women's needs. Having, in many cases, been educated within a hierarchical culture which assumes that health professionals know best, learning to become more open, prepared to question, and accepting of women's views has not been easy. I wonder, can obstetricians follow their example?

REFERENCES

1.   Maternity Services Advisory Committee. (1982). *Maternity Care in Action. Part 1. Antenatal Care.* (London: HMSO)

2. Maternity Services Advisory Committee. (1984). *Maternity Care in Action. Part 2. Care during Childbirth (Intrapartum) Care.* (London: HMSO)
3. Maternity Services Advisory Committee. (1985). *Maternity Care in Action. Part 3. Care of the Mother and Baby (Postnatal and Neonatal Care).* (London: HMSO)
4. Garcia, J. (1987). The role and structure of the Maternity Services Liaison Committee. *Health Trends, 19,*
5. National Audit Office. (1990). *Maternity Services Report by the Comptroller and Auditor General.* (London: HMSO)
6. Public Accounts Committee. (1990). *Maternity Services.* (London: HMSO)
7. Mason, V. (1989). *Women's Experience of Maternity Care – a Survey Manual.* (London: Office of Population, Census and Surveys, HMSO)

10

A politician's views

Renée Short

When I entered the House of Commons 28 years ago, backbenchers had some opportunity to monitor the activities of Government through a series of Estimates Committees, one for each spending department. There were nine members appointed, five from the Government side and four from the Opposition. I was appointed in 1965 to one of these Committees, monitoring the Health Department and was elected its Chairman. We had one Committee Clerk to help us to set up the enquiries and make arrangements for visits.

In 1967 the Estimates Committees were replaced by Expenditure Committees with 11 members and two or three staff, and we were able to appoint advisers from outside Parliament to help us with our enquiries. We were also able to travel abroad to look at good practice, having first got permission from the Steering Committee which consisted of the Chairs of all the Expenditure Committees. I was elected Chair of the Expenditure Committee monitoring the Departments of Employment and of Social Services – two large Departments to investigate.

After the 1979 election, the Expenditure Committees were pushed a bit further up the ladder and became Select Committees, with more resources for advisers for each enquiry and power to call Ministers as witnesses: they came before the Committee attended by three or four of their senior civil servants. We sat in public, with the Press present, and the attendance of Press and public at Select Committee hearings has increased.

Our first enquiry as a Select Committee was on perinatal and neonatal mortality. Professors Eva Alberman, Richard Beard and Osmond Reynolds were our advisers. After taking evidence in the House for some weeks we visited several hospitals involved in this highly specialized work.

At the conclusion of each enquiry we sat in private to consider the Draft Report and the recommendations to Ministers to be presented to Parliament; we were usually able to agree the Reports after two more sittings. In each Parliamentary Session several days are set aside to debate Select Committee Reports. The Steering Committee of Chairs would then meet to decide which Committee would have parliamentary time to debate a Report. We sat under the Chairmanship of Terence Higgins, Chair of the Treasury Select Committees whom we had elected as our Chair. At these meetings there could be two or three Chairpersons competing for Parliamentary time.

What is the raison d'être of our Select Committee system and how far does it fulfil that purpose? There are some parliamentarians who opposed Select Committees on the grounds that they took Members out the Chamber during debates and thus depreciated the importance of the proceedings in it. I do not agree with this view. Experience has shown that in any debate in the House the members of Select committees involved in those debates provide a core of informed views which has certainly improved the standard of Parliamentary debates. The public Proceedings and Reports of the Select Committees give MPs an insight into the actual machinery of Government and the way money is spent. It also enables the Opposition in Parliament to obtain vital information which they would certainly not be able to obtain otherwise.

Perhaps most significantly, the general public is given information and is thus much more aware of the machinery of Parliament and Government. As the Committees sit in public, members of the public can go and listen to the examination of witnesses and thanks to the Press and to the Reports issued by Select Committees they are able to learn something of Parliament's work. I always held a Press Conference when a new Report of my Committee was published. Our Reports on the Care of Children, on the Problems of Drug Dependence, on the Care of Mentally Ill and Mentally Handicapped in the Community, on Preventive Medicine, on Medical Education as well as that on Perinatal Mortality provided information not previously available, and led to a good deal of public pressure for change in these areas.

The continued existence of the NHS with its well-established principles of values and practice is now part of the national ethos, recognized and valued by the entire community. Any action that might be interpreted as hostile or destructive or likely to introduce unacceptable changes to the NHS, is bound to have immeasurable political consequences. The electorate may be volatile in a party-political sense, but when it comes to their basic interest, they usually find the courage to oppose and indeed campaign against Government policies. We have all heard about the reaction to the Poll tax as a result of which the Government decided to make concessions regarding their original proposals.

The present White Paper and subsequent legislation on the Health Service certainly originated in 10 Downing Street and reflect successive Tory Prime Ministers' political beliefs about competition and the dominating role of the marketplace. Should opposition to it become effective and inspire nationwide rejection, the Secretary of State would be told to think again and present fresh proposals that appear to be more acceptable to the professions and to the consumer.

This may involve prolonged consultation with the professions and result in delay as feasibility tests are carried out. There is also the question of funding; the professions cannot accept the basic aim of proposals, which is to keep resource funding from taxation within restrictive limits laid down by the Treasury. We are already behind all other industrialized countries in the proportion of Gross Domestic Product spent on our Health Service. The profession is faced with increasing costs as a result of the development of new methods of treatment and technology in medicine and surgery, and will not easily tolerate any reduction in research activity. Not only is the effectiveness of its day-to-day work dependent on increased clinical research but its professional standing world-wide depends on it. It seems to me that the White Paper proposals will inevitably lead to a severe restriction of research.

The political problem is largely one of timing. If the proposals and subsequent legislation are introduced now and are operative by the time of the next General Election their more serious effects will not have had time to become apparent, and the Government can go into battle assuring the electorate that 'the Health Service is safe in our hands'!

The art of presentation of policy is a matter that exercises Government greatly. Ministers are surrounded by experienced civil servants, skilled in the use of the enormous State machinery which is entirely at their disposal. They have at their fingertips a large amount of information which is not freely available to the Opposition or the public. The all-pervading secretiveness of our Governmental system ensures this.

Members of Select Committees can, on the other hand, endeavour to prise out some of this hidden knowledge from civil servants and Ministers who appear before them. Sometimes they succeed! This is their job and this is the way Parliament can exercise control over the Executive. When Select Committee Reports are published, members of the professions and voluntary organizations can then put pressure on politicians for changes they wish to see enacted. We must continue to campaign for the protection and proper resourcing of our Health Service.

General discussion II

Caroline Roach (Midwife, London)   Professor Beard's contribution starts off with a premise which, with all due respect, was actually presented some 20 or more years ago about the presumed advantages of hospital confinement. If we are looking to re-examine and to re-assess policy there is a great deal of evidence accumulated since which has called that premise into question. I would ask if we could perhaps move forward. We have to examine some of those old shibboleths and begin looking at the question anew from whatever professional or non-professional perspective we come.

Professor Richard Beard (Obstetrician, London)   The problem is that you present me as someone who has been a professional for many years and therefore perhaps I am reiterating old beliefs. This is not the case actually. I think you are wrong when you say there is a great deal of evidence to show that now we can tell the difference between high-risk and low-risk women in the antenatal period. Once we can do that, we will be in a completely different situation; the real problem, as anyone who works on a labour ward knows, is that a small proportion of women suddenly develop problems in labour that you cannot foretell.

Caroline Roach   What I said was that the premise that it was safer to deliver in hospital has been called into question. How we might make those distinctions is difficult; I think Professor Levene has offered some data which help us to see where we need to make the decisions. The premise of universal hospital delivery has been called into question and I think we have to move our discussion to that point.

Rupert Fawdry (Obstetrician, Milton Keynes)   Equally those who advocate out-of-hospital births have to prove that alternative forms of delivery are safer than in hospital. We were all glad to see the West Berkshire study which, although still hospital-based, presents an alternative way we could go.

The point about safety is paramount, but must be put into perspective. We would never go skiing or drive a car if safety was our only consideration. It has a place but we have to recognize that everything we do in life holds a risk. If a mother drives down the motorway with her children in the back of the car, she is taking a risk. We have to minimize that risk and we have to try to discuss with mothers the degree of risk they are taking, but can we really ban them from being allowed to decide to take a degree of risk?

I think it is depressing to say that midwives should be only concerned with the normal. The danger is that powerful obstetric professionals will push the frontiers of abnormality out further until there is nothing left that is normal. The people that come to me all have problems. The degree of the problems varies in severity; some I can deal with, others the midwife can deal with better.

Professor Malcolm Levene (Paediatrician, Leeds) I would totally disagree as far as risk is concerned; we have to identify risk and we have to minimize it. With reference to the newborn, at least the mother has the choice of evaluating the risks, the newborn does not have that choice. I am not arguing necessarily that all babies have to be born in hospital but whatever structure you put on this process, you have to ensure that it is as free from additional risk as possible. Nothing is risk-less, but we do have to minimize those risks. I think it is totally unacceptable to say that there is room for avoidable risk in whatever structure you set up, as far as delivering babies is concerned.

Professor Beard I think it is very easy for Mr Fawdry to talk about the risk that he is prepared to allow his mothers to take and other obstetricians will not. Before you do that, you have got to define what you mean by risk-taking; that is a very tricky area, particularly nowadays.

Rupert Fawdry I have never persuaded anyone to have a home delivery but I do not think I have the right to dominate their decisions.

Myra Farnworth (National Childbirth Trust Teacher and Tutor) We are all concerned with the question of safety and I would like to encourage us to use the available data. There is evidence concerning the issue of safety at home compared with hospital. From my understanding of the evidence, there is no evidence to suggest that even with a high-risk woman, home is statistically a less safe place to be.

Professor Beard You cannot make that assertion. High-risk women are not allowed to be randomized into home delivery as against hospital. Once you design that sort of project, then you can start to say you have got good data.

Beverley Beech (Association for Improvement of Maternity Services)   I must take issue with Richard Beard on some of the statements he has made. He said that we have to demonstrate that the alternative to hospital care is safer. I do not recall that your profession ever demonstrated in the first place that hospital care was safer when you were pushing to introduce it for everybody. You quoted the Peel Report and the Short Report and others; none of them produced any evidence that what they were proposing was going to be beneficial to all women. Electronic fetal monitoring, which the Short Report actually proposed for every single woman in this country, has now been shown to be a less useful technology and one that the Americans are going to abandon as a routine procedure. You said that you will not allow women to take the risk. Who are you, or anyone else to allow? We are in control of our bodies and our babies and we should be allowed to make the decisions. Unfortunately there are too many professionals who seem to think they have a right to allow a woman to do certain things and I think that is one of the fundamental problems within maternity care.

Professor Beard   Beverley Beech has not worked in my unit, but anyone who has knows that that is not at all the way in which obstetrics is practised; women are very much encouraged to have their own say. The maternity services need the support of everyone and we have got to work together for the future and not argue about old chestnuts as we are doing at the moment. Clearly I was not lucid enough when I spoke about influences on policy-making. I did not say whether I agreed with them or not, but they are a fact. Those are the reports which actually did dictate policy at that time. I was suggesting that there are now some new pressures that we need to look at and we need to have data.

Marjorie Tew (Medical Statistician, Nottingham)   Professor Beard stated that birth was safer in hospital. That means that birth was safer under obstetric management than under non-obstetric management. He also said that the onus is on those who challenge this to prove their case and that there are no data that they can prove it. Equally, of course, he must admit that there are no data on which the obstetricians can prove their case. Why should the greater obligation be on those who challenge than on those who assert this greater safety?

Professor Beard referred to randomized controlled trials; everybody realizes the possibility of any kind of randomized trial at this stage is quite out of the question. Therefore, what evidence do those who challenge his view have to produce to convince him of the soundness of the challenge? If you cannot use randomized prospective data, you have to use retrospective data from actual experience and when these data are analysed by risk groups, the rates are higher under obstetric management than under GP and midwifery care.

Professor Beard I think the last review I saw of home deliveries was by Alison MacFarlane and Campbell in 1978 where they came to the conclusion that the data showed neither home nor hospital deliveries had any benefit over the other; although hospital delivery had not been shown to be safer, it had not been shown to be less safe than other forms of delivery. I do think there is another way forward; it may not be a very popular thing to say in this gathering. With the advances in technology coming on, it is going to be possible to distinguish high-risk from non-risk more precisely. When we really get to that stage, it is reasonable to go back to Rupert Fawdry and say it looks as though although there is some risk involved, it is reasonably safe for you to have your baby at home. That is an obstetrician's view, but that I think is the way forward rather than trying to mull over these data which we will never get.

Marjorie Tew What I am challenging is that whatever the risk, as you identify it, the obstetric treatment does not make the outcome better than GP and midwifery treatment. I do not think you have got any evidence to show that is does.

Professor Beard Much of that is because the mother comes to us too late from the home in labour; remember, the perinatal mortality rate of those transferred in labour is very high.

Luke Zander (General Practitioner, London) I would like to consider ways we can ensure that we select appropriate policies of care. I was very encouraged by Professor Beard's statement that it is vitally important to use data and to undertake audit. The actual example you chose was whether the doctors in your unit would use a ventouse or a pair of forceps, in itself not a fundamental issue of controversy. However, we have to recognize that audit might change the basic direction in which the service is developing. How would your group have responded, for instance, to an audit on whether we should provide care for women in labour in the hospital or outside, an issue which would change the nature of working policies?

What was striking with Dr Kielty's contribution was that he was describing the feelings of general practitioners about the predicament they were in. What was striking, Professor Beard, in your contribution was that there was no sense of your personal involvement in the decision-making. We need to be prepared to accept that we have vested interests and feelings in the sort of programmes which we are pushing forward.

The consumer movement is unique in this sense because everybody knows mothers have a strong vested interest and that is often used as a reason to discount their particular contribution. We must not stand outside the arena and claim that only we are objective, and not suggesting policies which are supportive to our position.

If we can look at the neonatal example, we were told it would be criminal not to undertake a certain form of neonatal resuscitation. If the decision-making body was truly representative and multidisciplinary, it would need to look at what the effects would be on other aspects of the care system. We need to find a way in which we can have a much more non-hierarchical decision-making system, in which we can all play our part, contribute our individual input and then find a way whereby these differing perspectives can be sorted out in a much more multidisciplinary way.

Professor Levene I would like to take further Dr Zander's comment about resuscitation. I do not think anyone would argue that failure to resuscitate a baby is unacceptable in any obstetric unit anywhere in this country. What I contend is criminal, is that in some units there are people who are not trained in neonatal resuscitation. Who should do the resuscitation and how should it be done? There are teams of those who can resuscitate, wherever a baby is born; whoever delivers that baby needs to keep the baby alive until someone more experienced is available. There must be trained people everywhere babies are born, confident in resuscitating methods who are regularly retrained in resuscitation.

Luke Zander This particular argument about the safety of the mother and baby in the place of birth is now being used increasingly. One can see in the next decade a push to centralize more services and therefore one has a cost and gain equation. If all these facilities were available everywhere, that would be fine, but in fact the implication of what you say is now being used to redirect the way the maternity care is being organized.

Professor Beard What we are discussing here is power politics. Who makes the decisions? I have to say that we are never going to come down to some sort of flat world where everyone is absolutely equal. Of course, some obstetricians behave in an intolerant way. I could give examples about midwives too; what we really want is for all to get around a table. We try to do this locally, to say what are our roles in any particular activity and if we disagree about those roles we have it out, but in the end we must come to a decision. That is what we need to be doing today, not discussing the fact that obstetricians have too much power or that the NCT never gets off the ground.

Renée Short (Past Chairman, Parliamentary Select Committee on Social Services) Can I suggest to Mrs Beech that if she, or the organization to which she belongs, feels passionately about this problem, she could take some concrete action? All relevant organizations are perfectly entitled to write a testimony to the Select Health Committee of the House of Commons putting forward their points of view; the Select Committee will decide which witnesses to call to give oral evidence in the House of Commons. They will not listen unless you make them listen, so it is your job to present your written views and say that you would be willing to come and give evidence in public.

Sarah Roach (Midwife, Southampton) Mary Newburn's contribution highlighted something which can be remedied in the sickness that affects the maternity services. The Maternity Services Advisory Committee identified extremely clearly that it needed to be a team activity to make policies for the Maternity Services, and it suggested that Maternity Liaison Committees were set up. Lip service only has been paid to true team work and participation within those Committees; they are largely medically dominated while midwives and the consumer representative do not get a fair voice within the system. It is about time this was changed because really useful work could be done if we truly were able to act as a team.

Margaret Brain (President, Royal College of Midwives) We are looking at pregnancy care in the 1990s and how to advocate change. Although it is sometimes useful to look back and see what happened and why it happened, the purpose of this meeting is to look ahead. The power is swinging away from obstetricians towards midwives, who must declare a vested interest. It has been said there is no vision. The total midwifery model of care, with midwifery beds in every consultant and GP unit, is visionary and because it is so acceptable to everyone it will automatically go through.

If I could pick up the issue about the place of midwives in high-risk care, I tried to indicate that the high-risk woman and the low-risk woman require a different input from each of the professionals. As far as my own profession is concerned, the high-risk woman does require the social, emotional and educational support of a midwife to supplement the work of the obstetrician among women at higher risk.

Wendy Savage (Obstetrician, London) How can participation result in improved decision-making? We have a problem as professionals that we have spent many years acquiring knowledge and working hard all day and being called out at night. We feel threatened when that knowledge and experience is questioned by others who have not done this.

Renée Short made a very clear point about the importance of the Select Committees which enable the general public to get hold of information. Richard Beard showed how the North West Thames Regional Health Authority, using computer systems, is the only Region that was able to give any idea of what its Caesarean section rates were. In the States, there have been places where laws have been passed to make it possible for women to find out what the intervention rates are in particular hospitals. I would hope that in this country in the 1990s, such information would be freely available to women, and that we did not have to prise it out of reluctant Governments because it is our information, collected with our public money.

Another question concerns the perception of care. It is an insult to women to suggest that we care more about what happens to their babies than they do themselves. This raises women's hackles because, of course, they want to have a live, healthy baby and they will do anything to achieve that. We professionals have got to be absolutely sure that the advice we give them is based on good data and often it is not. What we have is a problem, which Mary Newburn illustrated in her description of what happened in Maternity Services Liaison Committees, that professionals find it very difficult to let go of their power; they feel weakened and threatened by doing so. In the 1990s we must find a way of really becoming a democratic society where people do have a voice and where people can sit down with professionals; unless consumers and professionals get together, we are going to be completely marginalized by accountants and experts in information technology.

We must go forward from this meeting with something positive. Too often the effect of women arming themselves with data has been to make the professionals retreat into their strongholds and refuse to talk. I do not know quite how to do it, but I am sure there are enough people here that we really could do it, if those of us in the professions could just relax a bit, to understand why it is that people like Beverley Beech get so angry when they hear people like Richard Beard speaking.

Professor Levene I find it extremely difficult to understand what it is I am raising people's hackles about. Are you suggesting that we should be doing a controlled study of resuscitation versus non-resuscitation for that is the only point that I have made? What obstetricians choose to do is clearly something for the profession in the wider sense together with the consumer. Is Dr Savage seriously suggesting that there is a doubt that resuscitation is ineffective or of no value?

Wendy Savage   No, I am not suggesting that. In your presentation, much of which was excellent, you did not once mention midwives. Who is the senior person present at the vast majority of deliveries in this country – the midwife. Why not train midwives properly to do the resuscitation instead of rotating GP trainees? There are ways that one could organize neonatal intensive care, with teams of young, enthusiastic neonatal care nurses who could go to a small hospital and deal with it. Who gives the care in neonatal intensive care units? It is the nurses who give the minute to minute care and those nurses are really skilled. If we are looking into the 1990s, we should be thinking about different models of care, but the attitude that came over from your presentation was that we, paediatricians, know how to organize things so that your babies will survive.

Professor Levene   I did not say at any time that only paediatricians should resuscitate babies; at least twice, I reiterated that anyone who is responsible for a delivery must be able to resuscitate the baby until more experienced or skilled care arrives. If you are a midwife, working in a unit that delivers between 1500 and 2000 babies a year, it might be once a year when you are called upon to resuscitate a baby. It is not possible for people to have up-to-date skills in advanced resuscitation in that sort of unit. If you think that all babies can be looked after by nurses in neonatal wards, then you are not living in the real world. We must have centralization of resources for the sickest babies and one has to plan across the board. Of all babies, 98% are going to be born in good condition, but 2% are not and 1% are going to be extremely ill; they will require intensive care which cannot be done in the ordinary District General Hospital without skilled neonatal intensive care facilities, requiring both nurses and doctors and equipment.

Professor Beard   I understand your longing to have an open debate with everyone being equal and saying their own thing, but we have been saying that for 20 years. Nothing happens about it because outside this room other things go on. The same old positions and relationships exert themselves. What I would like to see is everyone saying, it is the baby and the mother and her family that really interest us. We are all trying to do the same thing, that which is the best for them. Let us decide how we are going to do it within the confines of how we are working at the moment and with some proposals for the future. We cannot go back to an idealist but unrealistic democratic world.

Rosemary Scanlon (Stillbirth and Neonatal Death Society)   There are some success stories about working together between the voluntary sector and professionals. Ten years ago stillborn babies were taken away from their parents in the view that that was the best and kindest think to do. It was professionals and the voluntary sector working together that have changed that. There is now an understanding that if stillborn babies are born then the most useful thing that can happen is that a memory is created and that mothers can see and hold those babies if they wish. I think that it is important that the two sectors, working together, can use examples of good practice and can use what has happened successfully in order to take things forward. The Stillbirth and Neonatal Death Society (SANDS) decided two years ago to look at how to manage loss before 28 weeks. It set up a working party with representatives from all the relevant voluntary organizations and professional bodies. It was agreed that just looking at loss before 28 weeks was not sufficient. There were enough similarities between stillbirths and miscarriages to look at both situations together. There is still a mismatch of perception for parents who have a miscarriage; for them mostly, they have lost a baby, but for some professionals they have not necessarily lost a baby, they have lost a fetus. There are changes in the attitudes to the sufferers of miscarriage but in a recent conversation with a psychiatrist, he said 'I don't understand why women want to see their miscarriage. If I go to the toilet, I do not want to look at what I have just deposited in the toilet, why do woman want to look at their miscarriages?' That said something to me about his perception of it being a waste product.

If you look at the practice in hospitals about the disposal of babies that die before 28 weeks, there is an enormous amount of accumulating evidence that the hospital incinerator is still the usual method of disposal of these babies. So I think there is a challenge to policies for the 1990s in maternity services to look at what it means to parents below the 28th week and even below the 17th, 16th, or 15th week gestational limit.

How can this be got onto the policy agenda? What causes the continual mismatch of perceptions between the professionals and the families? How may this be changed and taken forward?

Professor Beard   When I wrote to *The Lancet* and suggested that the medical profession stopped calling miscarriage an abortion, almost overnight it occurred. I do think the profession is open to changes like this.

Professor Geoffrey Chamberlain (Obstetrician, London) The doctors and midwives in many units now are following what you started. We are looking upon those under 20 weeks as people in a continuum of reproduction. Someone does not become a baby just because he has passed 28 weeks. The work started in SANDS has flourished in the last few years.

Morris Mann (Public Health Consultant, Derby) In successful organizations, teamwork and team play do not just happen. People sit, think, plan and actually in some cases get in psychologists (you can see where this has worked in football teams for Sheffield United stayed in the First Division). I want to see obstetrics in this country stay in the first division.

There are other methods; the Dutch Government uses Strategic Choice Approach where the Government sorted out the ecology of midwifery. Are we aware of anywhere in England where we actually use these different decision-making processes? Have any of you any experience of formal team building or more sophisticated problem analysis and decision-making methods?

Charles Watters (Bristol and Western Health Authority) As a purchasing authority, I share Chris Ham's optimism about the split being an opportunity to listen to different voices and get a better overview of service needs and service provision. I wanted to ask Mary Newburn as an NCT representative, if she sees the purchaser/provider split as an opportunity for her organization and others to actually influence the way maternity services are bought?

Mary Newburn (National Childbirth Trust) There are certainly some people in the NCT who did think there was an opportunity, but it is quite clear that there are strong vested interests involved in decision-making. More so, I would argue from the evidence presented to me, now than was the case before.

We have not been terribly successful in influencing policy-making. I consider that multidisciplinary groups do not seem to have been used much. What seems to be important is training, needing to know with whom to talk and being prepared to engage in the debate.

Marion Hall (Obstetrician, Aberdeen) I want to comment on the question of ascertaining consumers' views and making sure they are represented in the policy-making. Firstly in my view, for health authorities to choose members of community health councils is corrupt. The second thing is that although we appreciate very much the well-articulated views of the pressure groups, such as the NCT, I think we have to make quite sure that we are also taking a systematic sampling of women's views. The recently produced OPCS manual by Beverley Botting is one which I think is a model in that respect. But that is not to say that the use of the pressure groups is not also of great value. To persuade the policy-makers, we need the pressure groups, but health authorities must also sample women's views.

Peter Kielty (General Practitioner, Harpenden) I think there is a very great opportunity for purchasers to influence what providers provide. Providers are not saying very much at the moment, maybe they will if we provoke them a little. The mothers with the pregnancies are of course the people who need the services and as their agent I am quite prepared, if my patients want things a certain way, to go and pressurize the purchasing authority until they get it. This is an enormous opportunity but will we seize it? Will we actually understand it? I do not think a lot of people have yet grasped how significant an opportunity it really is.

Rosemary Jenkins (Midwife, Royal College of Midwives) I would like to explore the way in which medical advance through research can involve the policy-makers and the resource implications. An example occurs in the neonatal field where we are probably fast moving towards a time when an artificial surfactant will play a significant part in the management of the very low birthweight baby. This is a marvellous medical advance which has taken some 8 or 9 years and now we are virtually at the end of the research period. It is going to have major implications on resources, because it will influence the number of baby days in intensive care units. At what stage in these processes do we have to talk to the policy-makers, the people who have the money? We need to indicate to them that something is on the cards that is going to have to shift resources.

Professor Levene There was a general and a specific question there. I think the general question is of great interest. You ask about a very expensive treatment, Surfactum®, but we could equally talk about antenatal steroid treatment which has been proven in a number of studies to have benefits in reducing the risk of respiratory distress in premature labour. Yet, how many obstetric units use it regularly? Certainly not as many as you would expect on the basis of this extremely well proven form of therapy. So you do not have to talk about expensive therapies only; we can talk about cheap ones.

Surfactant is a problem because it is expensive, costing about £400 per vial; a baby may need two, three or four treatments. It saves lives, but the babies do not have a shorter stay in the intensive care unit. There is an on-going dialogue both locally and nationally. Our Regional Health Authority and our District Health Authority are both aware that this is going to increase the cost and demand for neonatal intensive care. How are we going to answer the problem? We have not seen through that yet, although the immediate reaction is to say, we will work on the costing. Nationally, the British Association of Perinatal Medicine has put this as an item to discuss with the Select Committee on Health in order to have some national discussion as to how this new therapy will be funded.

Jilly Rosser (Institute of Child Health, Bristol) I would like us to have gone more into what actually does influence the making of policies, because it seems to me that we are going to have to look at that and understand it in order to change it. It has already been said that power comes into it, but what about the importance of ritual and feeling safe, however one likes to look at it. We all do feel safer doing things to women and we therefore have this system now whereby women are subjected tu enormous numbers of interventions, many of them not helpful and some of them positively harmful; it is going to be very difficult to climb down from that. We have enough evidence already from Iain Chalmers and others, to make enormous numbers of policy changes based on this available evidence, but how many policy changes are actually happening? Simple thinks like, is it useful to weigh women during pregnancy? Is a second routine ultrasound useful in pregnancy? This is more with midwives than obstetricians, when somebody comes to the antenatal clinic, of course we weigh them, because that is what you always did when somebody comes to the antenatal clinic. What are you going to do with your time? Giving iron to women who are not anaemic is positively harmful in antenatal care, but we carry on doing it; that is what we have always done and it makes you feel unsafe to stop doing it.

What about the recent research done on necrotizing enterocolitis in the newborn? I think this is interesting because it was a very convincing piece of research that reckoned that we could get rid of some 500 cases of necrotizing enterocolitis (including 100 baby deaths per year) by re-introducing milk banks, because preterm babies were dying from formula feeds. I would suggest to you that if there had been some wonder drug or wonder piece of equipment that was going to save 100 babies' lives, many neonatal units in this country would have adopted them immediately. However since the necrotizing enterocolitis is only to do with women's milk, it somehow does not fire the imagination of the policy-makers. That sort of thing is going to drag on for years and people are going to mumble about HIV and pasteurizers and 56 degrees while more and more babies continue to die from necrotizing entero-colitis. What is it about a certain piece of technology that excites us and makes us want to buy it and introduce it, while non-interventionist policies, of which milk is the perfect example, just go unheeded?

Professor Levene I think it is unfair to criticize paediatricians in the way that you have done. I cannot speak for all my colleagues, but it is generally accepted that breast milk is the milk that you start feeding preterm babies on. If there is no milk available you have to feed them on something. I would dispute the fact that this is the definitive study or that it is well proven. It is an interesting piece of information but it is not proven that breast milk is protective. Yesterday a baby died in my unit of necrotizing enterocolitis and the baby had had nothing but his mother's breast milk. It is not the only answer and we cannot over-simplify things to this extent.

I think the general points you make are excellent, but one has to not criticize paediatrics or obstetrics in general for what is done perhaps by individuals in individual units. Research is important but one needs to not necessarily believe every single paper that is written, one has to do overviews and I think the jury is still out on necrotizing enterocolitis. It is a very complicated condition which has many factors. Babies develop necrotizing enterocolitis without any milk at all, it certainly is not just milk.

Section 3
To what extent have research findings influenced policies?

11

Research findings and policy-making

Barbara Stocking

The way research influences policy and practice needs to be set in the context of how change comes about and the factors affecting it. This paper begins with some background as to what is known about why people change and adopt new or different practices; then looks at some of the evidence about research as an influence on these processes, and finally considers new ways of thinking about research if we want it to be used to bring about change.

THE CHANGE PROCESS

There is a considerable amount of literature on change, both from the perspective of innovation and the more general management literature on change as a management process. The innovation literature[1] shows that change moves through social systems as a fairly predictable process. Some innovations never become accepted. For others the rate of uptake will vary, but in general the 'S'-shaped curve in Figure 1 is followed. Innovation or change must be developed or promoted, but often such innovators are seen as maverick and are not highly respected in their professional or social system. Once the opinion leaders are convinced, others will follow, first those more oriented to change through to the most sceptical, leaving, at the end, a group of laggards who may never accept change.

The literature[2] suggests that the diffusion process follows the course of a point source phenomenon. The opinion leaders are those who go to national and international meetings. Back at home they adopt new practices and are then copied by their peers. It is possible to plot the dots

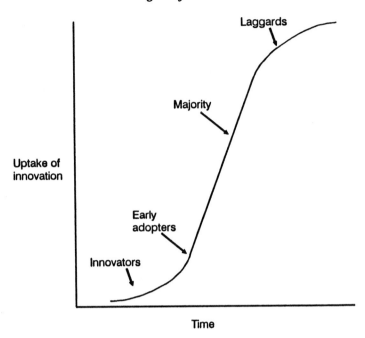

Figure 1 The rate of uptake of change. The innovators are characterized as 'venturesome'; the early adopters as 'respected'; the majority range from 'deliberate' to 'sceptical', and the laggards are 'traditional'

around a map as the opinion leaders accept an innovation, and the local spread which follows.

That may illustrate the change process, but which sorts of innovation are acceptable and which are not? Rogers highlighted five key characteristics of innovations which influence their adoption. He termed these characteristics relative advantage or loss, compatibility, complexity, trialability and observability[3].

The first, relative advantage, may be the place where research ought to figure. If a medical practice is shown to be more effective than another then that ought to give it relative advantage, although it is not quite so simple. A medical innovation may be perceived to have advantages or disadvantages well beyond the benefit to patient care; it may give security or reassurance to professionals; it may reduce time pressures; require new skills, or increase or decrease income, and so on. It has to be remembered that each individual with all his personal and environmental complexity will assess advantage in a quite personal, if implicit, way.

A fundamental stumbling block to adoption of a change is that it is incompatible with beliefs or working practices. Possibly, research findings do not have the expected impact because they are incompatible with long-held philosophies and practices. Changes in the environment may be necessary to alter something more fundamental before a specific new idea can be accepted.

Complexity is also off-putting. If a change requires the involvement of a large number of disparate people and actions, then the negotiations will be complex and individuals' prestige and influence may be affected. Change then will be difficult. An example is that of changing patient waking times in hospitals[4], in essence a very simple idea but one which turns out to be highly complex. To change waking times requires the involvement of virtually all staff in a hospital: day and night nurses, caterers, cleaners, doctors, and the various departments such as X-ray and physiotherapy where patients may be taken. It is not surprising then that change has been difficult, especially when it has been led by people such as ward sisters with relatively little power to influence other groups.

My own research has shown that introducing the most difficult, incompatible and complex changes has the more interesting results. Once the change is made it tends to stick. So many people have been involved and have needed to compromise and adapt their philosophies that there is no going back. The opposite occurs with the very simple add-on technologies. They may be adopted more quickly but once the product champion goes away practice drifts back easily to what it was before.

The final key characteristics of innovations are observability and trialability. Can you see the innovation in operation and can you try it out on limited basis? Though influential, these seem to be of lesser importance than the others. Innovators certainly recognize the need for observability, often running open-house sessions, and the champions may take teams of people to see an activity in operation to show that it is possible. This does not always have the desired effect, especially if the observed site has additional resources. Trialability also has negative aspects. Sometimes trial of ideas in a limited way may help persuade people to adopt them; for complex changes, however, building up the commitment for a large once-and-for-all change may help make it stick.

I have found that the ability to adapt something to local circumstances and not to have too much precision about exactly what should be done can help its adoption. This is something of a problem for research findings which are often seen as emanating from somewhere else. It is also an issue when research findings are built into guidelines and standards. Without local modification they may not be at all acceptable.

RESEARCH AND PRACTICE

How people change is a complex mixture of themselves, their environment and the nature of change itself, and it is therefore not surprising that the implementation of research findings in policy and practice is not straightforward. Overall, we know that research has had a surprisingly limited effect on practice. Apart from the complexity of the change process we need to look at some of the other factors which may present problems to implementation.

First, there is evidence that research has very little impact on the diffusion of new technologies and practice, because the results are often not available at the time people are making decisions about a practice or technology. There are exceptions to this rule. Sometimes there are concerns about risks of a procedure and people may be prepared to move slowly until studies are available identifying risk. I think this was the case in the early days of amniocentesis[5]. Sometimes a whole infrastructure needs to be present to support the development, and before health authorities are willing to make the investment they will look for guidance which may give time for research results to become available. In recent years some governments, notably in Sweden and The Netherlands, have become clearer about the need for evaluation before decisions are made about the diffusion of expensive medical technologies. Both countries required evaluation of the lithotripter for kidney stone treatment before agreeing policy. In the case of Sweden the county councils waited for the evaluation results before purchasing other than the experimental machine; however, although the resulting policy was followed for a short time it has now been broken[6].

While central governments and financing bodies may step in where major technologies are concerned for economic or ethical reasons, on the whole they do not become involved in clinical practice. In those cases the doctors and other health professionals involved need to be convinced of the need for evidence if they are to take part in or wait for the results of evaluations. Chorionic villus sampling (CVS) is interesting in this respect. In some countries there was a conviction that CVS was self-evidently better or not as good as amniocentesis. This led to differences between countries in their willingness to take part in trials. Even in the countries which have been involved in trials, the practice has spread beyond the trial centres, once again showing how difficult it is to suspend judgement.

If evaluation is a weak influence on early diffusion, that does not mean it cannot have an effect subsequently: perhaps altering the rate of diffusion, for example, stopping increased use or making clear the circumstances on which a practice is appropriate. There are some exam-

116

ples too where late evidence has dramatically reduced the use of a technology. Studies in the USA showing the lack of benefit and, in fact the poorer outcomes, for patients taking certain drugs led to the almost complete abandonment of some oral antibiotic drugs and a cholesterol-lowering drug. Fears about malpractice have been a significant factor in these examples, however[7].

Apart from issues of timing, the case is often made that research does not answer the questions nor meet the needs of the doctor or nurse in practice[8]. The trials may be of questionable quality, but even if good they may have relevance only to a specific group of patients, or not be applicable in ordinary conditions of use. It is difficult to know how much truth there is in these criticisms and how much it is a matter of just not believing the evidence. In any case the meta-analysis work now being undertaken should help elucidate some of the issues.

Overall, the evidence for research, particularly clinical trials, influencing practice is limited. This evidence was summarized a few years ago by the office of Technology Assessment[9].

APPROACHES TO INFLUENCING PRACTICE

Some researchers believe that if they simply publish their work in the appropriate journals it will have the desired impact. Many others now understand that there is a lot more to the dissemination of ideas, and also a great deal of work to be done if these ideas are to be accepted and result in changes in practice. A number of more or less explicit approaches have been tried.

Information feedback

A number of researchers have tried to feed back to practising professionals, usually doctors, information of two sorts: research evidence about a particular procedure, and feedback on the individual's practice compared to a group or compared to a standard.

While information is necessary for change the results showed it is not sufficient. 'Passive' information giving does not result in change, it needs to be linked into a wider strategy[10].

Guidelines, standards and peer pressure

There is some evidence[11] that local agreement about a practice, perhaps as a result of the development of national guidelines, can lead to change if there is peer pressure or some means of group audit. Ensuring guidelines are adhered to may require a great deal of persistence by local leaders because of the movement of junior doctors or simply because individuals become less interested in the process. It remains to be seen whether the new focus on medical audit will be successful in achieving changes in practice, assuming of course the agreed changes themselves were based on scientific evidence.

External incentives

From the USA in particular there is considerable evidence that practice can be manipulated by the reward system. This seems to be happening in the UK too, specifically the GP contract where, for example, it is claimed that payments for reaching targets for immunizations have led to a significant increase in immunization rates. Once again, though, the rewards ought to be based on scientific evidence but, regrettably, often they are not. The benefits of screening for the over 75-year-olds in the GP contract are still in dispute. There are significant drawbacks to using financial incentives to change practice. Apart from the fact that it may develop a philosophy where financial reward becomes more important than patient benefit, it does not necessarily encourage doctors to be more sceptical about their practice and look for evidence.

Consumer power

There is certainly evidence in the field of perinatal care that consumer power has managed to alter practice. However, there have been very limited attempts to harness this consumer power to ensure evidence-based practice, though perhaps the involvement of consumer groups with the UK CVS trials is an important such development.

Using the change process

Perhaps the most interesting work on how to get evidence used in practice is being undertaken at McMaster University in Canada[12]. These workers undertook a national consensus conference on the use of Caesarean sections, and this in itself was based on a rigorous analysis of the scientific evidence. More significantly, they also looked hard at all the literature on bringing out change and have adopted strategies based on that knowledge. For example they have carefully identified local 'influentials', brought them together and taken them through all the literature and conclusions. They have also got the commitment of those influentials to taking the ideas back and they have been provided with material to use. This is just one strategy and they are experimenting with others. The studies have shown that change of practice is more effective with influentials than audit[13]. Some of the early results are a little disappointing, though, in that even these approaches may not be producing change. It may be that each individual change, for example, trial of labour for women who have had previous Caesarean sections, needs considerable analysis itself, looking at all the factors influencing behaviour.

MAKING RESEARCH INFLUENCE PRACTICE

If that analysis seems somewhat disheartening I do believe that there are steps we can take to do better. The prerequisites are that we understand better the processes of change, and that we analyse in detail the changes we want to bring about, to understand what factors influence current behaviour and what needs to be done to achieve change.

It is important that the climate of opinion is right. For example if the changes goes against widely accepted beliefs it may be more important to first change the overall climate of opinion than to battle on with the specific change.

Next a variety of means can be used to get the message across and to exert pressure. An idea needs to come from different places before it gradually seems to be what you have always believed. Written material is one source, but what people say to each other is much more influential. We do need to identify and enlist the opinion leaders, both at national and at local level. We need to use pressure on doctors, particularly from other health professionals and from patients – and there is a communications strategy in itself to get good information to patients.

In the NHS of 1991 we also must not forget the power of purchasers. We need to make sure they have much better access to scientific information and persuade them to use it in their purchasing specifications and in negotiations with the providers.

For any individual change we need to assess what the stumbling blocks are and try to remove them. For example, if there are real personal, organizational or financial disincentives for a change, we may need to alter these first. Individuals may feel they cannot undertake a new procedure because they are not trained, for example.

Finally, we have to make it possible for people to own the change themselves. This is particularly difficult for scientific evidence which is coming from elsewhere. We need to find ways to encourage local people to decide how to incorporate changes based on evidence in their practice.

This list may seem a major challenge, but without it the funds spent on research may often be wasted and patients may continue to receive inappropriate care.

There is an even broader challenge. It may be that even with quite complex strategies it is going to be very hard to achieve change in practice unless we can make a fundamental attitude shift – namely establishing that wherever possible practice should be based on sound scientific evidence. This requires substantial work in undergraduate and postgraduate medical education. It is the fundamental challenge to us all.

REFERENCES

1. Rogers, E. (1983). *Diffusion of Innovations*, 3rd edn. (New York: New York Free Press)
2. Hagerstrand, T. (1967). *Innovation Diffusion as a Spatial Process*. (Chicago: University of Chicago)
3. Rogers, E. (1983). *Diffusion of Innovations*, 3rd edn. pp. 210–40. (New York: New York Free Press)
4. Stocking, B. (1985). *Initiative and Inertia*. (London: Nuffield Provincial Hospitals Trust)
5. Reid, M. (1991). *The Diffusion of Four Prenatal Tests Across Europe*, pp. 8–19. (London: King's Fund Centre)
6. Kirchberger, S. (1991). *The Diffusion of Two Technologies for Renal Stone Treatment across Europe*. (London: King's Fund Centre)
7. Finkelstein, S.N., Schectman, S.B., Sondik, E.J. and Gilbert, D. (1981). Clinical trials and established medical practice: two examples. In Roberts, E.B., Levy, R.I., Finkelstein, S.N., Moskowitz, J. and Sondik, E.J. (eds.) *Biomedical Innovation*. (Cambridge, MA: MIT Press)
8. Herxheimer, A., Zentler-Munro, P. and Winn, D. (1986). *Therapeutic Trials and Society*, pp. 17–20. (London: Consumers Association)
9. Office of Technology Assessment. (1983). *The Impact of Randomized Clinical Trials on Health Policy and Medical Practice*. (Washington DC: US Congress)
10. Mugford, M. (1991). Effects of feedback of information on clinical practice: A review. *Br. Med. J.*, 303, 398–402
11. Fowkes, F.G.R. (1985). *Strategies for changing the use of diagnostic radiology*, King's Fund Project Paper No. 57. (London: King's Fund)
12. Lomas, J. (1990). Promoting clinical policy change: Using the art to promote the science in medicine. In Anderson, T.F. and Mooney, G. (eds.) *Economic Issues in Health Care: The Challenges of Medical Practice Variations*. (London: Macmillan Scientific and Medical Press)
13. Lomas, J., Enkin, M., Anderson, G.M., Hannah, W.J., Vayda, E. and Singer, J. (1991). Opinion leaders vs. audit and feedback to implement practice guidelines. *J. Am. Med. Assoc.*, 265, 2202–7

12

The content and process of antenatal care

Marion Hall

THE CONTENT OF ANTENATAL CARE

Research areas relevant to policy-making

Biomedical research can help to describe the normal universe, the boundaries of pathology, and the extent to which biochemical or biophysical measurements vary from the normal before or during clinical manifestation of problems. However, there are many pitfalls in the interpretation of such research. Because pregnancy lasts for 40 weeks, cohort studies where serial measurements are made on the same women are expensive, and may not contain large enough numbers to include women with relatively rare clinical problems, such as abruption or severe intrauterine growth retardation. It is quicker and cheaper to substitute studies with cross-sectional measurements where results on groups of women at different gestations are combined to provide a picture of change in advancing pregnancy, and the temptation to do this is not always resisted. Another problem is that, for example, low values of components in body fluids may be misinterpreted as deficiency, or small fetal size as intrauterine growth retardation.

However, the main problem with biomedical research is that even when it has been clearly shown that a biochemical or biophysical test has a close relationship to a serious clinical problem, the next stage of careful evaluation of whether in practice the utilization of this test actually benefits the mother or the fetus, is often eschewed in the rush to develop the exciting new innovation. This is discussed well by McKinlay[1], who described the following seven stages in the career of an innovation: promising report; professional adoption; public accept-ance; standard procedure and observation; randomized controlled trials; professional denunciation of randomized controlled trials, and finally, erosion and discreditation leading to replacement. This is unfor-tunately a recurring phenomenon. My conclusion is that biomedical research has had too great an effect on policy, or at least on practice.

Epidemiological research can of course also be of great value in describ-ing both normal and complicated pregnancy, and the maternal charac-teristics and behaviours associated with these. The results of studies showing recurrence risks of pregnancy problems, such as pregnancy hypertension, smallness for gestational age or preterm labour, are wide-ly used in antenatal care. However, the understanding of the predictive value of previous obstetric history has been advanced by the use of longitudinal, as opposed to cross-sectional, analysis, pioneered by Bak-keteig and Hoffman[2], using the Norwegian Birth Registry. A great deal of work has been done on the development of weighted scores to combine multiple risk factors to predict pregnancy outcome, but doubt has now been cast upon their value[3]. The problems that arise with the practical application of either single or multiple risk factors are firstly, that there may or may not be an appropriate intervention, especially for social problems[4], and secondly, that the intervention may do more harm than good when applied to the false positives which occur with all risk factors in current use.

Sociological research has added a new dimension to our understanding of potential advantages and disadvantages of methods of organizing care for pregnant women. This can of course take many forms: enlight-ening us about beliefs and attitudes to pregnancy itself, to tests and procedures, on the psychological costs of awaiting results[5] and about the need for information and support. Of course, the sociology of health service providers[1] and policy-makers is also of interest.

Health services research should determine the content of antenatal care for women in a developed country such as the UK. This would ideally consist of a marrying together of the results of epidemiological, socio-logical and biomedical research to identify the problems of pregnant women, and then interventions would be offered which have been fully evaluated by randomized controlled trials. Only by such evaluation can it be certain that the treatment will do more good than harm. Testing and screening can be similarly evaluated, separately from the interven-tions.

Economic assessment is also essential to discover which of the effective screening programmes and/or interventions are providing best value for money.

Application of research findings to practice

How does current antenatal care measure up? Very little economic evaluation has been done, and the large variation in the number of visits recommended and performed in different European countries[6] suggests that factors other than rational scientific assessment determine levels of care. Very little information is routinely collected about the amount of care provided, but there is plenty of indirect evidence that, in practice, the results of randomized controlled trials have had less influence on practice than they should. An exhaustive analysis is not possible here but some interesting examples may be considered.

Routine haematinic administration

Meta-analysis[7] of studies concerned with the routine administration to well-nourished women of iron and folic acid show no benefit in respect of any pregnancy complication, and there is no evidence that the rise in haemoglobin and folate levels is an advantage. Nevertheless, haematinics are almost universally prescribed, suggesting that doctors are indeed susceptible to advertising.

Routine ultrasound scanning

Ultrasound is not known to be harmful, and there are a considerable number of situations in which a scan is helpful in early pregnancy, such as confirmations of doubtful gestation, of intrauterine pregnancy if there is a risk of ectopic, or of a live fetus where there has been a threatened miscarriage. Remarkably few randomized controlled trials of routine scanning have been done, and there is no clear evidence of better health outcomes, though there is a suggestion that induction for postmaturity may be performed less often. Nevertheless, a booking scan is almost always offered, and indeed now demanded by women. There is also no evidence that a routine third trimester scan for growth reduced mortality or morbidity, though it can detect growth disorders in most cases.

Possibly adverse consequences of routine early or late scans are anxiety about unexplained or insignificant findings. It must be emphasized, however, that although evidence of benefit from routine scanning is scanty, there is little evidence of harm. However, it is a pity that such an expensive intervention with major capital costs for developing technology, and revenue costs for training and service provision, has not been more systematically evaluated.

Assessment of low risk

The current UK arrangements for confinement mean that a very small proportion of women are delivered in the primary care sector. Comparison of some recent European studies[8–14] shows that the proportion booked for primary care varies from 47 to 87%, indicating that differing criteria are in use. Contrary to what would be expected, the centres booking more women for primary care transfer fewer to specialist care during the antenatal period. Again, though the antenatal transfer rate varies from 10 to 30%, the centres transferring most women antenatally seem to need to transfer just as many in labour as those with low antenatal transfer rates. This indicates that antenatal care is not proving very successful in foreseeing problems that might arise in labour, though women are led to believe that it can do this. Is this because the results of research are not being incorporated into care, or because antenatal care is simply rather ineffectual?

Routine care to detect pre-eclampsia

Because hypertensive disease in pregnancy is a major cause of maternal mortality, frequent visits are justified by the need for regular blood pressure measurement. Using the number of women attending the clinic as the denominator, traditional care was shown to be of low productivity[15] and a more rational schedule proposed. This was implemented in Aberdeen[16] and the number of visits reduced. This did not prove to be dangerous as the proportion of cases diagnosed for the first time in labour actually fell.

Further work in Aberdeen[17] has confirmed, using the number of undelivered women in the population as the denominator, that traditional care has a very small chance of detecting pre-eclampsia[16] sufficiently severe that delivery is needed within two weeks. However, our impression is that the pattern of care in Aberdeen (administered largely by GPs) has reverted to something nearer the traditional pattern. The system has a great inertia, and women's views may play a part in this.

RESEARCH AND THE PROCESS OF ANTENATAL CARE

There have been consistent reports[18] of unsatisfactory care, especially in hospital clinics; well validated methods of ascertaining women's views are now available[19] and medical and midwifery audit will be essential in self-regulation. New initiatives in the provision of team midwifery care, providing much better continuity are to be welcomed. The question of how continuity can be achieved in the care provided by general practitioners, who do not undertake intrapartum care, needs to be addressed.

CONCLUSION

It is doubtful whether the content or process of antenatal care in Britain could be described as meeting the requirement of the House of Commons Health Committee, that the most appropriate and cost-effective care of pregnant women should be achieved. It is to be hoped that matters will improve in the 1990s.

REFERENCES

1. McKinlay, J.B. (1981). From 'Promising Report' to 'Standard Procedure': Stages in the career of a medical innovation. *Millbank Memorial Fund Quarterly (Health and Society)*, 59
2. Bakketeig, L.S. and Hoffman, H.J. (1981). Epidemiology of preterm birth: results from a longitudinal study of births in Norway. In Elder, M.G. and Hendricks, C.H. (eds.) *Preterm Labour*. (London: Butterworths)
3. Alexander, S. and Keirse, M.J.N.C. (1989). Formal risk scoring during pregnancy. In Chalmers, I., Enkin, M. and Keirse, M. J.N.C. (eds.) *Effective Care in Pregnancy and Childbirth*, pp. 345–65. (Oxford: Oxford University Press)
4. Bryce, K. (1990). Social and midwifery support. In Hall, M. (ed.) *Baillère's Clinical Obstetrics and Gynaecology. Antenatal Care*, pp. 77–88.(London: Baillière Tindall)
5. Marteau, T., Kidd, J., Cook, R., Johnston, M., Michie, S., Shaw, R.W. and Slack, J. (1988). Screening for Down's Syndrome. *Br. Med. J.* 297, 1469
6. Blondel, B. (1986). Antenatal care in the countries of the European Community over the last twenty years. In Breart, G.M., Buekens, P., Huisjes, H.J., McIlwaine, G. and Selbmann, H. (eds.) *Perinatal Care Delivery Systems*, pp. 3–15. (Oxford: Oxford University Press)
7. Mahome, K. and Hytten, F. (1989). Iron and folate supplementation in pregnancy. In Chalmers, I., Enkin, M. and Keirse, M.J.N.C. (eds.) *Effective Care in Pregnancy and Childbirth*, pp. 301–17. (Oxford: Oxford University Press)
8. Chng, P.K., Hall, M.H. and MacGillivray, I. (1980). An audit of antenatal care: the value of the first visit. *Br. Med. J.*, 281, 1184–6
9. Street, P., Gannon, M.J. and Holt, E.M. (1991). Community obstetric care in West Berkshire. *Br. Med. J.*, 302, 698–700
10. Young, G. (1987). Are isolated maternity units run by general practitioners dangerous? *Br. Med. J.*, 294, 744–6
11. Marsh, G.N. and Channing, D.M. (1989). Audit of 26 years of obstetrics in general practice. *Br. Med. J.*, 298, 1079–80

12. van Alten, E., Eskes, M. and Trefors, O. (1989). Midwifery in the Netherlands. The Wormeveer Study: selection, mode of delivery, perinatal mortality and infant morbidity. *Br. J. Obstet. Gynaecol.*, 96, 656–62
13. Ris, M. (1986). Obstetrical care in the Netherlands. The place of midwives and specific aspects of their role. In Breart, G.M., Buekens, P., Huisjes, H.J., McIlwaine, G. and Selbmann, H. (eds.) *Perinatal Care Delivery Systems*, pp. 167–77. (Oxford: Oxford University Press)
14. Smith, L.F.P. and Jewell, D. (1991). Contribution of general practitioners to hospital intrapartum care in maternity units in England and Wales in 1988. *Br. Med. J.*, 302, 13–16
15. Hall, M.H., Chng, P.K. and MacGillivray, I. (1980). Is routine antenatal care worthwhile? *Lancet*, 2, 78–80
16. Hall, M.H., MacIntyre, S. and Porter, M. (1985). *Antenatal Care Assessed.* (Aberdeen: Aberdeen University Press)
17. Hall, M.H. and Campbell, D.M. (1992). Cost effectiveness of present programmes for detection of asymptomatic hypertension in relation to the severity of hypertension and proteinuric hypertension. *Int. J. Technol. Assessment in Health Care*, in press
18. Garcia, J. (1989). *Getting Consumers' Views of Maternity Care.* (London: HMSO)
19. Mason, V. (1989). *Women's Experience of Maternity Care – a Survey Manual.* (London: HMSO)

13

The basis of a midwifery team: continuity of carer

Caroline Flint

In 1988 the Association of Radical Midwives sent a letter[1] to all Community Health Councils, branches of the Royal College of Midwives, the Association for the Improvements of Maternity Services, the National Childbirth Trust, Midwifery Schools and selected members of Parliament which said:

> 'We support any scheme in which a woman has the opportunity of getting to know a small number of midwives who will provide her care throughout pregnancy, labour and the postnatal period.'

The Association was becoming concerned at the number of 'Midwifery Teams' which were planned at the time where the basic principle behind such schemes appeared to have been forgotten: mainly continuity of carer. Note that I use the words 'continuity of carer' rather than 'continuity of care', because in the power games we play with parents we twist words so much that they become meaningless; and for many people 'continuity of care' has become synonymous with 'continuity of advice' rather than the continuity of personnel that women have been requesting from us for many years.

No woman has ever asked to be looked after by a 'Midwifery Team'[2]; women have been asking to be looked after during labour by someone who has given them antenatal care and whom they have been able to get to know, as the following reports, from various sources, demonstrate:

> 'She would like, if it were possible, to have someone around during her labour who had given her some antenatal care'[3].

127

'I think this is what women complain about most: they do not have continuity of care which they want very much during their antenatal visits but certainly during labour and delivery.'
'We recognize the difficulties of providing continuity of care throughout pregnancy and labour but consider that a measure of it can be attained by better organization'[4].

'There is an almost complete absence of continuity of care and each time she attends a woman sees different, anonymous faces'[5].

'It is important that the woman should be able to build up a relationship of trust with the staff she meets, and efforts should be made to involve the same group of staff at each visit'[6].

'I was more relaxed because my midwife was with me.'
'By and large it is the midwife who makes or breaks a happy delivery.'
'These women enjoyed labour – they were given choice, they were attended by midwives they liked.'
'My labour was a truly delightful experience attended by professional people that I regarded as friends'[7].

'It has been suggested to us that women should have the same midwife to attend them in labour as in the antenatal period. We consider this continuity of care to be an ideal aim and it may be possible in some circumstances'[8].

'Plan effective continuity of care – women should have the opportunity of building up a relationship with one doctor, one midwife'[9].

'Mothers would like antenatal, delivery and postnatal care to be provided, as far as possible, by the same people. Again and again, letters expressed the anxiety that arises when seeing a different doctor at each visit to the antenatal clinic, and at being delivered by total strangers – sometimes two different shifts of total strangers if a woman had a long labour'[10].

'Good communications between parents and the medical staff were helped where women saw the same doctor and midwife regularly. Most mothers saw different people at almost every antenatal visit and were delivered by total strangers. While full of praise for the care they received, many women wished they could have had more continuity of care through pregnancy and beyond'[11].

'I feel that everybody would benefit from knowing the midwife who delivers them. I found this to be extremely important when

in labour. I would have been much more nervous and scared if I hadn't known and trusted my midwife.'
'It would be nice if you could see the same midwife all through your pregnancy then during labour.'
'The same midwife should follow the patient from clinic to delivery to postnatal ward and hopefully to her home afterwards'[12].

WHAT ACTUALLY INFLUENCED POLICIES?

There has been some research into continuity of care given by a team of midwives[13–18]. In many ways the research findings have acted as fuel to justify the setting up of teams of midwives in an attempt to provide women with a semblance of the continuity for which they have been asking.

The 'Know Your Midwife' scheme was a randomized controlled trial, undertaken at St George's Hospital, London, between 1983 and 1985, in which 1001 women who were deemed suitable for midwife care were randomly assigned to two groups. In one group each woman was looked after by a team of four midwives, who provided antenatal, labour delivery and postnatal care to the women, who were able to get to know the four midwives. They knew that one of the four midwives would be with them during labour. Their levels of satisfaction and feelings of being in control of the situation were markedly greater than those of the control group, who received normal fragmented care from a mixture of hospital midwives and doctors[12]. Barbara Stocking suggests that it is publicity and hearing the same thing from many different sources that influences policies. Many surveys of women's views of their maternity care have shown that women are asking for continuity of carer, but the medical and midwifery professions did not start to hear what women were saying until midwives began to take up the same message. Once there was proper research evidence to back up women's wishes, action was initiated.

SETTING UP A MIDWIFERY TEAM

I have had the privilege of involvement in the setting up of four different types of midwifery teams: the St George's Hospital 'Know your Midwife' scheme, the Kidlington team in Oxford, the Riverside midwife teams and the West London Hospital teams. I would like to share with you some of the experiences I have gathered along the way.

Some teams are set up with the desire to give women continuity of carer, some are set up to ensure a more efficient deployment of midwifery staff. Both appear to improve job satisfaction amongst midwives but not necessarily to improve continuity of carer as far as women are concerned. However, when women are cared for by midwives who are happy in their work it would be supposed that some of this pleasure would rub off on the women.

Ideas for a team scheme have to come from the workers; it is no use imposing a structure from above and expecting the midwives to go along with it. They have to do the work, they need help and support, but their ideas and suggestions must be paramount otherwise resentment will ensure that the scheme is doomed from the start. However well organized and highly motivated the staff appear to be, change is extremely painful and demands so much from people that if a scheme is imposed on then it will simply be too hard to do, and they will sabotage it.

The organizers need to be aware that each team develops differently. The off-duties will be different, the approach will be different, even the way the midwives look, the clothes they decide to wear, will be different[19,20]. Each team will develop a team identity.

Never underestimate how painful, disorientating and difficult change is. The midwives involved need support, workshops, teaching in how to support each other, affirmation of how well they are doing and recognition of how painful this period is.

THE DOOMED PILOT SCHEME

It is my impression that pilot schemes are extremely vulnerable and my advice would be not to set them up. If there is a desire for a team scheme it should be set up throughout the health authority or hospital.

The vulnerability of a pilot scheme arises because all the eager beaver midwives apply for the midwifery team posts so that the other staff feel threatened by the excellence of the care given by the team and resentment erupts. The team is showing up the mediocrity of normal care. The team is scapegoated; everything was better before the team started, the unit ran more smoothly, the water in the taps was hotter, the linen arrived on time, the pharmacy was more efficient, the students were more respectful, the patients were more compliant. The team knits together to arm itself against the antagonism of the other staff, and has no other team to provide support to or gain support from. One mishap happens – a baby is stillborn, or there is a near miss – and the team is disbanded.

Also it is the starting up of a team which is difficult; having embarked upon it once, even the most superhuman midwifery manager would baulk at having to go through the setting up process twice or several times.

FACTORS WHICH MILITATE AGAINST TEAM MIDWIFERY

Inertia is a considerable factor; the problems of change are so great that only the bravest and most committed will embark upon change. Team midwifery at its best changes real fundamental issues: the balance of power shifts from the professionals to the mother. The women become stronger and more powerful; they feel that it is their right to refuse to have medical students in the room when they are in labour, they expect to be involved in decision-making and refuse to be bossed about. All this makes them more difficult for the majority of midwives and doctors, accustomed to compliance, to deal with.

GPs find team midwifery extremely threatening. It was the local GPs who prevented a midwifery team scheme starting in Manchester some four years ago. In the Riverside community there have been several attempts by GPs to sabotage the scheme either by not telling women about the scheme or by sending them elsewhere for their care. This seems surprising when it is obvious that GPs themselves care about, and provide continuity of care to, most families throughout life. Why would they have a problem about a group providing continuity of care throughout pregnancy and labour?

The reason may be financial: pregnancy care represents about £200 for the GP. If he or she has 50 pregnant women a year going through the surgery that represents £10 000 towards the annual financial turnover. GPs are afraid that if midwives carry out more and more antenatal care this proportion of their annual earnings is under threat.

Another reason is the pleasure of seeing pregnant women. GPs see sick, depressed, terminally ill patients all day; their pregnant patients represent a pleasant interlude for them, and they enjoy caring for healthy pregnant women.

Along with the 'Know Your Midwife' research a survey was carried out on 577 women who were receiving shared care with their GPs[12]. The women met the same criteria as the randomized groups and were given the same questionnaires as the randomized groups with a few extra questions relating to their shared care. Women who received shared care had short waiting times when attending for antenatal consultations; 65.4% waited less than 15 minutes. A total of 85.4% were satisfied with their antenatal care but their satisfaction with the care was not as great as the women receiving care from the group of four midwives, the 'Know Your Midwife' team.

When women who had received shared care came to labour they appeared to miss out. As would be expected, the obstetric outcome was very similar to that of the women in the control group in the main study, but their feelings about their labours were very different. They felt less well prepared for labour than women who attended the hospital ante-natal clinic throughout pregnancy and much less prepared than women who were cared for by the 'Know Your Midwife' team. They did not feel that they had managed as well as the other two groups of women, especially the women looked after by the 'Know Your Midwife' team. Six weeks postnatally, only 17.4% felt that they had been very much in control during labour compared with 41.9% of the 'Know Your Midwife' women. They also felt less well prepared for looking after a baby.

This is the only piece of research to examine women's feelings following shared care with GPs. As this is so commonly practised, it is suggested that it should be examined further. The research report suggests that GPs should be more willing and be made more welcome so that they feel able to come into labour wards to see their patients, simply on a social basis, because women are asking for someone they know to be with them during labour and delivery. Even if GPs don't have the expertise to deliver or to conduct the labour, the fact that they are there and that the women know the GP is important to women.

Consultant obstetricians can also try to prevent midwives from working in teams. They are afraid that midwives will become too autonomous and that this may challenge their dominance in the labour ward. Most team schemes are hedged about with several restrictive policies which ensure that the obstetricians have the final say in what is happening.

For example, in the 'Know Your Midwife' scheme, the notes of each woman had to be shown to a senior registrar before she could be included in the randomization, despite very strict criteria. Interestingly one senior registrar always found more 'abnormalities' than the researcher did, in fact she stopped taking notes to him quite early on otherwise she would not have had anyone deemed 'suitable for midwife care' at all. The senior registrars she used had to be carefully selected.

With the Riverside midwife teams the same criteria apply and all notes have to be discussed with an obstetrician; there is no realization that midwives are quite content with normal, low-risk women. The sense of being deprived of a job is very strong in the medical profession. One wonders what the root of this fear is; could it be that if women were left to midwives very few would need medical help?

Other midwives often sabotage suggestions for setting up team schemes: they are afraid of change; they do not have the energy to change; or they are retiring soon so they would rather not bother. Energy levels are very low within the NHS, and in some Units may be too low to enable anyone to initiate a scheme.

PROBLEMS WITH MIDWIFERY TEAMS

The responsibility felt by the team midwives is much greater than that felt by most midwives. When a midwife is out in the community making decisions it can feel extremely hard. Unlike her hospital colleague, she does not have someone else to confer with or a doctor close at hand to refer to. The doctor available to her probably has not done any obstetrics since his medical student days and is not as up-to-date as she is herself. With the extraordinary system of supervision of midwifery and the over-zealous disciplinary system many midwives rightly feel under threat at all times.

People making clinical decisions will inevitably, if they have been practising for any length of time, make a misjudgement, a clinical mistake. Even though the decision in theory was the correct one, in practice it may be the wrong one and a disaster may occur. The supervisor of midwives must understand the implications of making clinical decisions, and the doctors should appreciate that the midwives are making clinical decisions based on a different philosophy from the medical one: namely that labouring women are going through a normal process until it is shown to be abnormal, rather than the philosophy that childbirth is only normal in retrospect. Then midwives are safe, not from criticism or debate, but from censure. On the other hand if the supervisor does not understand this and the doctors are ready to be vindictive, the midwife can end up before the Local Supervising Authority and the Investigating Committee, in danger of being struck off from her profession. All midwives are aware that the stakes are high, and many are aware that it is just a matter of luck whether they happen to be dealing with a sympathetic supervisor or not.

The autonomy of team midwives is heavy for midwives to bear when they are used to abrogating responsibility to doctors or more senior midwives. Menzies[21] pointed out how in the nursing model responsibility is pushed further and further away from the bedside and so diffused that no-one feels the weight of it. With team midwifery this is not the case, the autonomy of the practitioner can be a heavy burden.

Being on call is extremely stressful for team midwives. It has been known for team midwives to be unable to sleep when on call because they have been waiting for the bleep to go off and have been afraid that they might not hear it. Other midwives feel constrained by the bleep:

they feel unable to go out when on call and dislike the fact that they cannot drink when they are on call. Most midwives on call dislike the possibility of being called at any time, and not knowing whether they will have six hours sleep or six minutes.

The intensity of feeling is also a shocking corollary of working with a group of women that you are able to get to know. As one midwife said to me after having delivered a stillborn baby: 'Caroline, I've delivered stillborn babies before, but I've never cried about them, I've never had vivid dreams about them, I've never felt so sad before'. My response was: 'But you've never known the parents well before – this time the real magnitude of the grief has hit you because you love the parents, you were anticipating that baby too, you can't be untouched by this, it means too much'. Conversely, although the sad times are much sadder, the happy times are much happier. The joy and intensity of feeling that goes with being a midwife, is wonderful in this situation.

THE FUTURE

It is clear that we have to provide continuity of care for women[19,20,22]. We have to set up more teams of midwives, more midwives need to have their own caseloads. Midwives can work with the woman's GP. He has provided continuity of care until now so the woman should be encouraged to see him once or twice during pregnancy, and he should be encouraged to visit her during labour. However, if he cannot manage that, it is of no consequence if she has with her a midwife she has been able to get to know during pregnancy.

The role of the consultant obstetrician should become just that: someone to be consulted when obstetric expertise is needed. Otherwise, pregnancy should be perceived as a normal human function that women and midwives can happily manage on their own.

REFERENCES

1. Association of Radical Midwives. (1988). Letter to all Community Health Councils, Royal College of Midwives branches, Association for the Improvement of Maternity Services, National Childbirth Trust, Midwifery Schools and selected MPs, 15th May.
2. Flint, C. (1986). A Different Face Each Time. *Nursing Times*, May 14th
3. Micklethwaite, P., Beard, R. and Shaw, K. (1978). Expectations of a pregnant woman in relation to her treatment. *Br. Med. J.*, 2, 188-91
4. House of Commons Social Services Committee. The Short Report. (1980). *Second Report: Perinatal and Neonatal Mortality.* (London: HMSO)

5. Kitzinger, S. (1981). *Change in Antenatal Care*. (London: National Childbirth Trust)

6. Maternity Services Advisory Committee. (1982). *Maternity Care in Action. Part 1: Antenatal Care*. (London: HMSO)

7. Boyd, C. and Sellers, L. (1982). *The British Way of Birth*. (London: Pan Books Ltd)

8. Royal College of Obstetricians and Gynaecologists. (1982). *Report of the RCOG Working Party on Antenatal and Intrapartum Care*. (London: RCOG)

9. Ong, Bie Nio. (1983). *Our Motherhood*. (London: Family Service Units)

10. (1983). Birth in Britain. A Parents special report. A survey of 7 500 women's views. *Parents*, **92**

11. (1986). Birth: 9000 Mothers Speak out. Birth Survey 1986 – results. *Parents*, **128**

12. Flint, C. and Poulengeris, P. (1987). *The 'Know Your Midwife' Report*. (London: 49 Peckarmans Wood, SE26 6RZ)

13. Cushing, J. (1989). Resume of findings. Evaluation of the Rhondda Know Your Midwife Scheme. The First Years Deliveries. Director of Midwifery, Clinical Practice and Research, 6th Nov. (Personal communication)

14. Haire, D. (1981). Improving the outcome of pregnancy through the increased utilization of midwives. *J. Nurse-Midwifery*, **26**, 5–8

15. Kowalski, K., Gottschalk, J., Greer, B., Watson, A. and Bowes, J. R. (1977). Team nursing coverage of prenatal – intrapartum patients at a University Hospital. *Obstet. Gynecol.*, **50**, 116–19

16. Oakley, A. Rajan, L. and Grant, A. (1990). Social support and pregnancy outcome. *Br. J. Obstet. Gynaecol.*, **97**, 155–62

17. Runnerstrom, L. (1969). The effectiveness of nurse-midwifery in a supervised hospital environment. *Bull. Am. Coll. Nurse-Midwives*, **14**, 40–52

18. Slome, C., Wetherbee, H., Daly, M., Christensen, K., Meglen, M. and Thiede, H. (1976). Effectiveness of certified nurse-midwives. *Am. J. Obstet. Gynecol.*, **124**, 177–82

19. Association of Radical Midwives. (1986). *The Vision – Proposals for the Future of the Maternity Services*

20. Royal College of Midwives. (1987). Towards a Healthy Nation. (London: RCM)

21. Menzies, I. E. P. (1970). *The Functioning of Social Systems as a Defence Against Anxiety*. (London: Tavistock Institute of Human Relations)

22. Chalmers, I., Enkin, M.W. and Kierse, M.J.N.C. (eds.) (1989). *Effective Care in Pregnancy and Childbirth*. (Oxford: Oxford University Press)

14

Place of birth

Gavin Young

'A man convinced against his will
Is of the same opinion still.'

The proportion of births occurring at home in England and Wales has dropped from 85% in 1927 to under 1% in 1985. Over the same period, the perinatal mortality rate has dropped from 60.8 to 9.8 per 1000 total births. Some would argue that no further evidence is required; that the UK policy of centralizing birth in specialist hospitals is entirely vindicated by the contemporaneous fall in perinatal deaths.

Childbirth has increasingly been viewed as dangerous and frequently requiring immediate medical help. This view is shared by lay people and professionals alike. However, within the history of childbirth it is very recent. In 1936 the British College of Obstetricians and Gynaecologists stated that:

'Adequate hospital provision for all cases could only be made at great expense: the results of domiciliary midwifery do not warrant such expenditure'[1].

What brought about the dramatic shift in views? Was it scientific evidence?

One major influence was the creation of the NHS. Expectant mothers could afford to deliver in hospital, and many wished to do so. The number of hospital obstetricians increased in parallel. Penicillin became available, as did anti-tuberculous drugs and hospitals came to be seen as benign, problem-solving institutions.

A significant series of Government-commissioned reports between 1959 and 1984 made the following recommendations:

'Sufficient hospital...beds for 70% of all confinements to take place in hospital'[2].

137

'We think that sufficient facilities should be provided to allow for 100% hospital delivery. The greater safety of hospital confinement for mother and child justifies this objective'[3].

'An increasing number of mothers be delivered in large units; home delivery be phased out further'[4].

'The practice of delivering nearly all babies in hospital has contributed to the dramatic reduction in stillbirths and neonatal deaths and to the avoidance of many child handicaps'[5].

These reports, largely based on opinions of hospital-based professionals, have now almost achieved their ultimate aim: all women in the UK delivering in large specialist hospitals. The shift to hospital care over the past 40 years is one of the most fundamental changes in health care. Was there evidence to support this change?

EVIDENCE OF GREATER SAFETY OF HOSPITAL BIRTH?

Three kinds of evidence provided support for the idea that specialist hospital care was safer. As already mentioned, the fall in maternal and perinatal mortality coincided with an increase in deliveries under specialist care. Secondly, transfer of patients from home or 'isolated GP units' was associated with high perinatal mortality rates[6] and finally, the personal experience of many obstetricians who saw, and remembered vividly, some of those patients transferred with problems. This third category is of little value. One would not examine an orthopaedic ward in Zermatt to discover if skiing is an experience of acceptable safety.

Behind the evidence lay, and still does lie for many, the unshakeable belief that hospital must be safer. Common sense would indicate that it must be safer to deliver where full facilities are available to cope with any possible mishap during or after delivery. Yet, common sense tells us that the sun goes around the earth. Galileo found clear evidence to the contrary, but despite the evidence, many in authority stuck to their previous belief.

Archie Cochrane doubted the evidence for centralizing maternity care:

'It is surprising how successive committees have been content to accept trends as something God-given which must be followed, instead of demanding a more rigorous analysis of causality'[7].

Is there now a need to undertake such an analysis? I believe there is.

First, and most importantly, there is powerful anecdotal evidence from consumer bodies such as the National Childbirth Trust, the Maternity Alliance and the Association for Improvements in the Maternity Services, that the centralization of care, the closure of small isolated units and the difficulty in obtaining a home birth are resented by many women. Such anecdotal reports are supported by consumer surveys[8,9]. If there is evidence that present policy is disliked by the consumer, this should motivate a closer scrutiny of that policy and the evidence on which it was based.

Secondly, making available the full range of obstetric facilities may well be a waste of resources when the majority of women can deliver without medical assistance.

Thirdly, the centralization policy is still active. Home births and isolated units are still threatened. If existing policy continues, any opportunity to study possible alternative forms of care will be lost. Is there evidence that centralization is not the only, or the best, option?

EVIDENCE AGAINST CENTRALIZATION

Figures for home births are difficult to interpret. A direct comparison with hospital should not be made as planned home births are, by and large, to low-risk women. Hospital tends to be the place of delivery for women predicted to be at high risk, for example diabetics or those with a breech presentation. Nonetheless, it is reasonable to examine the figures for home births to see if it can be considered 'safe enough'. It is only if one option is to be allowed to exist that one must make a comparison. Paradoxically, the UK has virtually taken this stance, despite not making a comparison. Home birth figures have been misinterpreted. The Cardiff births survey revealed that by 1979 the number of unplanned home births in that survey exceeded births planned to occur at home[10]. This shift has a huge impact on the apparent lack of safety of home birth. A survey of all home births in England and Wales in 1979[11] showed that the perinatal mortality rate for planned home births (67% of total) was 4.1 per 1000 total births but for births not booked anywhere (3%) the rate was 196.6 per 1000. Births booked for hospital but which took place at home (21%) had a perinatal mortality rate of 67.5 per 1000. In 9% of home births intended place of delivery was not known. Unfortunately, this survey was not able to discover the outcome for women moved from home in labour. This remains a very difficult area of research, though Dutch evidence is that such transfers raise the perinatal mortality rate very little. Nonetheless, the survey showed a very low rate for women delivering at home.

Isolated GP units have been closed down on the grounds of lack of safety. They came in for particular attack in the Short Report[4]. Such units are still being threatened with closure this year. What evidence exists regarding their safety?

Before looking at the evidence it is necessary to understand the nature of these units. By 'isolated' it is meant that the units are geographically distant from specialist help. For the women who use them they are not isolated: it is the specialist help which is isolated. By 'GP' it is meant that the medical back-up for the unit is provided by GPs. It might be more appropriate to call these hospitals 'rural midwifery units'. Most will not have facilities for general anaesthesia nor for Caesarean section and will, therefore, offer few extra facilities beyond those available at home.

Nonetheless, the great majority of women served by such units choose delivery there rather than at home or in a specialist unit (unpublished data, available from the author). It is not clear why, and it would be a useful piece of research to discover how a woman reaches her decision concerning choice of place of delivery.

A postal survey of all isolated GP units (131 in number) in England and Wales in 1977 (89% response rate) found the perinatal mortality rate to be 5.1 per 1000 total births[12], including the cases transferred in labour. My own much smaller but more detailed survey of the isolated unit at Penrith in Cumbria[13], found a rate of 4.7 per 1000 for all women starting labour in Penrith.

The above evidence conflicts with the opinions given to government committees by hospital specialists. The opinion of the Royal College of Midwives (RCM) was also against such units, and it is interesting that the RCM appears now to have moved away from the 'only the centre is safe' view. A variety of studies from other countries, that is, Finland, Canada and New Zealand, has been examined by Roger Rosenblatt[14]. All the studies suggested that outcomes for low-risk obstetric populations may be better in less technologically intensive settings.

It is this last finding that makes many (including women using maternity services) have doubts about the policy of centralization. A 5-year prospective study[15] of home births in Essex from 1978 to 1983, using matched controls under specialist hospital care, found no perinatal deaths in either group but found the induction rate to be twice as high in the hospital group, and an increased second-degree tear rate, despite a higher episiotomy rate. This finding, of a higher intervention rate in low-risk women when under specialist care, was repeated in a comparison of women booked under GP and midwife care in the integrated unit in Oxford as against a similar low-risk group booked under specialist care on the same unit[16].

The most exhaustive study in the UK, analysing perinatal mortality rate by place of birth, was Marjorie Tew's analysis of unpublished data from the British Births 1970 survey[17]. An attempt was made to overcome the bias that specialist hospitals delivered difficult cases, by giving each woman an antenatal and labour weighting for risk, known as a 'prediction score'. Using these scores, Tew found significantly lower perinatal mortality rates in the GP units and at home as compared with specialist hospitals for all levels of risk, except the very highest where the difference did not reach significance level. This study has been criticized because it may reveal that the prediction scores were invalid. However, until recently there has been almost no evidence pointing in the opposite direction to Tew's findings.

A recent paper from Bath[18] matched low-risk women in Bath with like women booked to deliver in rural GP units. This study found the perinatal mortality rate in the central unit to be 2.8 and in the rural areas 4.8 per 1000 total births. However, this included deaths before labour began. It was not, therefore, solely a study of the safety of birth in different units. Perinatal mortality rates after the onset of labour were 0.9 and 1.5 per 1000 respectively, which does not reach significance level.

This study has been given wide publicity and needs examining. It is in essence a study of low-risk urban Bath women compared with low-risk rural women. Most of the perinatal deaths occurred before labour and it is not clear in what ways these might have been avoided if the rural units had not existed. It is unlikely that specialist care would have affected these antenatal deaths. The chance of a baby surviving after an antepartum haemorrhage decreases with distance from the place of Caesarean section, that is rural women will fare less well whatever the facilities available. The perinatal mortality rate in the integrated, central, GP unit was zero by intended place of delivery at the time of onset of labour, or the time of diagnosis of intrauterine death.

The evidence overall about safety and place of birth in the UK suggests that home and isolated units are as safe as consultant care for the women who choose such care. There is not now a large enough number of births in these settings for a proper comparison to be made. Campbell and MacFarlane's review of the evidence up to 1985 included this comment:

'It would have been possible to mount such a trial in the 1960s or early 1970s when substantially more women were giving birth at home and it is unfortunate that such an opportunity was missed by the successive committees who made recommendations about the place of delivery'[19].

The Netherlands is now the only country in the developed world where such evidence can be made available. In 1988 36% of Dutch women delivered at home. The perinatal mortality rate in the Netherlands is the same as in the UK. This information itself raises major doubts about the justification for the British policy of centralization which is, however, shared by all other developed countries.

THE DUTCH EXPERIENCE

A very detailed study of 7980 women booking with midwives in and around Wormeveer, just north of Amsterdam, between 1969 and 1983 was published in 1989[20]. This study involved 92% of the nulliparous women and 79% of parous women in the catchment area. Of these women, 75% had midwife-only care, either in a small maternity unit or at home. The perinatal mortality rate for these women, including those transferred in labour, was 2.3 per 1000 total births. The national figure over this period was 14.5 per 1000. Though this study, as in all the previous studies cited, is not a randomized controlled trial, it does show that the great majority of women can give birth safely away from specialist care. It is unlikely that the perinatal mortality rate would have been better had they delivered under specialist care and there might have been more intervention. (The Caesarean section rate in the midwife-only group was 0.4%.) Regional perinatal mortality rates in the Netherlands do not correlate with the degree of hospitalization[22].

The UK is not the Netherlands, yet the Dutch evidence cannot be ignored or, rather, it should not be. In the event, it has been ignored and it is striking even now, how those who make decisions about place of birth, whether they are members of government committees making recommendations to the Department of Health, specialist obstetricians deciding health authority policy or GPs advising their patients, can continue to be so adamant that birth away from specialist care, particularly at home, is unsafe.

PERINATAL MORBIDITY

There is no evidence that perinatal morbidity would be influenced by place of birth. Obstetric technology appears unable to affect the incidence of cerebral palsy. A 5-year follow-up of the Dublin trial found no difference in the incidence of cerebral palsy whether there had been continuous electronic fetal monitoring or intermittent auscultation[22]. A review of two large studies, from Western Australia and the National Collaborative Perinatal Project in the USA, came to the conclusion that in less than 10% of cases of cerebral palsy was intrapartum asphyxia a factor[23].

CONSIDERATIONS OTHER THAN SAFETY

If the evidence about safety of birth away from specialist care is equivocal, are there any other factors upon which evidence has a bearing? Recently, cost has been the reason put forward for the proposed closure of rural units. The economics of maternity care are discussed in another chapter, but it is worth explaining here that the apparent cost-effectiveness of a form of care is very dependent on the use made of it. Thus, if a small unit is underused it will become uneconomic. Providing community midwifery cover for occasional home births is expensive when hospitals are still staffed for 99% of births.

Evidence about intervention has already been presented. This difference in behaviour between specialist and primary carers has been recognized by women and may explain much of the anecdotal evidence in favour of primary, midwife and GP care, as well as the evidence from surveys[8,9].

PSYCHOSOCIAL FACTORS

It is reasonable and desirable to provide maternity care of a kind which women want unless there is clear evidence of lack of safety. That a particular form of care is chosen, and is therefore more comfortable for the woman, may be important. Unfortunately, evidence about the effect of separating women from familiar surroundings and known carers at the time of birth is minimal, though there is animal evidence of harmful effects[24].

Mammalian evidence points to an overriding need for the pregnant animal to feel safe when she gives birth. In humans it is likely that the pregnant woman will be the best person to decide where she will feel most safe, having been given available evidence about possible places of birth. Her carers cannot decide for her where she will feel most safe. There is evidence of the great importance of maternal psychological state on the outcome of labour. A study from a hospital in Guatemala showed that lay support could halve the length of labour, compared with that of women left alone in labour[25].

CONCLUSION

The overall evidence about safety and place of birth shows no significant differences in outcome, maternal mortality, perinatal mortality or morbidity, between primary care units and specialist hospitals.

It would be unthinkable that road travel between London and Edinburgh should be phased out because the railway industry believed it was a safer way of travelling between the two cities. Yet, in effect, a similar process has occurred with maternity care in the UK. Campbell and MacFarlane[26], after the most extensive search of maternity statistics in the UK, conclude:

'There is no evidence to support the claim that the safest policy is for all women to give birth in hospital'.

and

'The policy of closing small obstetric units on the grounds of safety is not supported by the available evidence'.

The final words of their study are depressing:

'Perhaps the most persistent and striking feature of the debate about where to be born, however, is the way policy has been formed with very little reference to the evidence'.

One is left wondering what evidence would be required to persuade those who make policy to change it.

As with the choice between road and rail travel, choice of place of birth does not depend solely on safety. Cost may be important. In the USA cost leads women to have 'out of hospital' births[27]. In the UK, evidence about cost in different settings, as with safety, is equivocal. However, the evidence about consumer preference is less equivocal. UK policy about place of birth needs re-examining, especially by a government that purports to encourage choice in maternity care.

RECOMMENDATIONS

Because of the evidence, or because of the lack of it as regards safety, it is possible to suggest changes to present UK policy:

(1) It should be more widely recognized that place of birth has only a minor part to play in affecting perinatal mortality. Therefore, rather than limiting choice of place of birth, it would be more productive to research the causes of congenital malformation, preterm labour and intrauterine growth retardation.

(2) Remaining isolated rural units should be retained where women wish them to be.

(3) Pressure against home births should be eased.

(4) Low-technology birth centres should be built, attached to, but having a separate identity from, the specialist unit. These could be staffed by midwives, possibly with GPs as medical support. (There

is evidence that many integrated GP units suffer from loss of identity and enthusiasm as compared to attached units[28].)

(5) Selection for birth in primary care settings should be based on Dutch criteria[29], as these are based on very much greater experience of birth in such settings.

(6) The training of midwives and GPs should be changed to allow them to be able to undertake safely most care at birth, as at present large areas of the UK have no one competent to help a women deliver her baby.

(7) Research should be undertaken into which factors affect a woman's choice of place of birth.

(8) Research should be undertaken into how psychological and social factors affect the progress and outcome of labour.

REFERENCES

1. British College of Obstetricians and Gynaecologists. (1936). *Outline of a Scheme for a National Maternity Service.* (London: BCOG)
2. Ministry of Health. (1959). *Report of the Maternity Services Committee.* (Chairman, Lord Cranbrook). (London: HMSO)
3. Standing Maternity and Midwifery Advisory Committee. (Chairman, Sir John Peel). (1970). *Domiciliary Midwifery and Maternity Bed Needs*, p. 54. (London: HMSO)
4. Social Services Committee. (Chairman, Mrs Renée Short). (1980). *Second Report: Perinatal and Neonatal Mortality*, p. 27. (London: HMSO)
5. Maternity Services Advisory Committee. (1984). *Maternity Care in Action: Part 2: Care during Childbirth*, p. v. (London: HMSO)
6. Hobbs, M.S.T. and Acheson, E.D. (1966). Perinatal mortality and the organization of obstetric services in the Oxford area in 1962. *Br. Med., J.* 1, 499
7. Cochrane, A.L. (1972). *Effectiveness and Efficiency: Random Reflections on the Health Service*, p. 63. (London: Nuffield Provincial Hospitals Trust)
8. National Council of Women of Great Britain. (1990). *Are We Fit for the 90s?*, p. 5. (London: National Council of Women, N1 8JU)
9. Taylor, A. (1986). Maternity services: the consumer's view. *J. R. Coll. Gen. Pract.*, 36, 157–60
10. Murphy, J.F., Dauncey, M., Gray, O.P. and Chalmers, I. (1984). Planned and unplanned deliveries at home: implications of a changing rate. *Br. Med. J.*, 288, 1429–32
11. Campbell, R., MacDonald Davies, I., MacFarlane, A. and Beral, V. (1984). Home births in England and Wales, 1979: perinatal mortality according to intended place of delivery. *Br. Med. J.*, 289, 721–4

12. Cavenagh, A.J.M., Phillips, K.M., Sheridan, B. and Williams, E.M.J. (1984). Contribution of isolated general practitioner maternity units. *Br. Med. J.*, **288**, 1438–40

13. Young, G. (1987). Are isolated maternity units run by general practitioners dangerous? *Br. Med. J.*, **294**, 744–6

14. Rosenblatt, R. (1987). Perinatal outcome and family medicine – refocusing the research agenda. *J. Fam. Pract.*, **24**, 119–22

15. Shearer, J.M.L. (1985). Five year prospective survey of risk of booking for a home birth in Essex. *Br. Med. J.*, **291**, 1478–80

16. Klein, M., Lloyd, I., Redman, C., Bull, M. and Turnbull, A.C. (1983). A comparison of low-risk pregnant women booked for delivery in two systems of care. *Br. J. Obstet. Gynaecol.*, **90**, 118–22

17. Tew, M. (1985). Place of birth and perinatal mortality. *J. R. Coll. Gen. Pract.*, **35**, 390–4

18. Sangala, V., Dunster, G., Bohin, S. and Osborne, J. (1990). Perinatal mortality rates in isolated general practitioner maternity units. *Br. Med. J.*, **301**, 418–20

19. Campbell, R. and MacFarlane, A. (1986). Place of delivery: a review. *Br. J. Obstet. Gynaecol.*, **93**, 675–83

20. van Alten, D., Eskes, M. and Treffers, P.E. (1989). Midwifery in the Netherlands. The Wormeveer study; selection, mode of delivery, perinatal mortality and infant morbidity. *Br. J. Obstet. Gynaecol.*, **96**, 656–62

21. Treffers, P.E. and Laan, R. (1986). Regional perinatal mortality and regional hospitalisation at delivery in The Netherlands. *Br. J. Obstet. Gynaecol.*, **93**, 690–3

22. Grant, A., Joy, M. O'Brien, N., Hennessey, E. and MacDonald, D. (1989). Cerebral palsy among children born during the Dublin randomised trial of intrapartum monitoring. *Lancet*, **2**, 1233–6

23. Nelson, K.B. (1989). What proportion of cerebral palsy is related to birth asphyxia? *J. Paediatr.*, **112**, 572–3

24. Naaktgeboren, C. (1989). The biology of childbirth. In Chalmers, I., Enkin, M. and Keirse, M.J.N.C. (eds.) *Effective Care in Pregnancy and Childbirth, Vol. 2*, pp. 795–805. (Oxford: Oxford University Press)

25. Klaus, M., Kennell, J., Robertson, S. and Sosa, R. (1986). Effects of social support during parturition on maternal and infant morbidity. *Br. Med. J.*, **293**, 585–7

26. Campbell, R. and MacFarlane, A. (1987). *Where to be Born? The Debate and the Evidence*, p. 58–9. (Oxford: National Perinatal Epidemiology Unit)

27. Acheson, L., Harris, S. and Zyzanski, S. (1990). Patient selection and outcomes for out-of-hospital births in one family practice. *J. Fam. Pract.*, **31**, 128–36

28. Smith, L.F.P. and Jewell, D. (1991). Contribution of general practitioners to hospital intrapartum care in maternity units in England and Wales in 1988. *Br. Med. J.*, **302**, 13–16

29. Kloosterman, G.J. (1984). The Dutch experience of domiciliary confinements. In Zander, L. and Chamberlain, G. (eds.) *Pregnancy Care for the 1980s*, pp. 115–25. (London: Royal Society of Medicine and Macmillan Press)

15
Neonatal intensive care

Richard Cooke

Neonatal intensive care has been described as an ongoing experiment, and it is the area of paediatrics which in recent years has been most subject to advance and change based on the influence of research findings.

When looking at clinical practice there are three areas which research findings might alter. Firstly the situation where nothing makes very much difference. The patient will either recover or die despite what is done. Although doctors do not like to recognize it, a substantial part of daily practice falls into this category. It is the category where there is most variation in practice from one doctor or unit to the next, and the main function of research is to help one discard useless or ineffective therapies in order to make life simpler.

A second area is where the actual management is absolutely critical to the survival or good outcome of the infant. Often the effects of management are so dramatic that there is little argument over how the patient should be managed and a relatively small role for new research findings. Unfortunately such situations are relatively uncommon.

A third area can be termed, the grey area in between, and it is here that research findings are most useful. An intervention may not have an 'all-or-none' effect but nevertheless may contribute usefully to the improvement of mortality or morbidity. Most new developments in medicine fall into this area, for example drugs to prevent periventricular haemorrhage in the newborn.

Trials of drugs such as ethamsylate, vitamin E and indomethacin, all show a modest effect in reducing haemorrhage in particular high-risk groups. Centres using such drugs have not managed to abolish the condition altogether. Only by the use of carefully designed clinical trials have the useful effects of such drugs been demonstrated.

If we are to examine ways in which research findings are translated into neonatal practice, we should perhaps look at the stages in life when a young doctor might take these findings on board.

It might be supposed that the seeds of appreciation of research findings should be sown whilst he is still at medical school. Here the student has only a few weeks to learn the principles of the practice of obstetrics and neonatal care. Only the most basic principles can be put across, and of necessity this must be done with a didactic approach in order to save time. Research techniques are not seen as having any immediate clinical relevance, although attempts are made at teaching them by exposing students to statistical methods and epidemiology. This exposure is usually at a separate stage of teaching and not usually integrated with clinical practice, in particular neonatal practice.

After qualifying, the young doctor moves through the pre-registration house year and into a senior house officer post. These posts comprise an apprenticeship in the traditional sense, and at this stage the resident learns neonatal medicine as it is practised. Most young doctors find that their main objective at this stage is simply to get through the day. It is difficult to take anything but an uncritical approach and in fact any other is not usually appreciated by his seniors.

Having survived those first years as a junior, the doctor may graduate to registrar and senior registrar status, and at this stage be mostly concerned with postgraduate examinations. He learns to read journals, begins to attend conferences and even involve himself in his own research. This should be the golden opportunity for acquiring an appreciation of research findings and of how they might be applied to daily practice.

Unfortunately, the budding researcher is often ill-prepared and guided, and he may drift into the 'white swan' approach to medical research. This approach tackles the hypothesis 'all swans are white' by looking for white swans. The more white swans he finds, the more he feels that he has confirmed his hypothesis. Unfortunately only the finding of a black swan will contribute any new useful information to ornithology. The idea of collecting similar cases and recording them persists in journal titles such as the 'Archives of Disease in Childhood'.

There also persists a belief that there are two entirely different forms of research, clinical and laboratory which use entirely different methods and approaches. Even if a doctor does perform research and becomes competent in a certain area, he may well find this is narrow and of relatively little application in his daily work, reinforcing the concept that research is not relevant on a day-to-day basis. Once at consultant level the new doctor may pick up relatively little in the way of new developments and research, and settles easily into a daily routine of clinics and ward rounds, and if he is lucky a little golf!

We should perhaps consider how research findings could be disseminated to the medical and nursing profession. The use of medical journals would be the first and most obvious route. Unfortunately their sheer number makes it difficult for busy staff to find those papers and reports most appropriate to their needs. There is a tendency to read reviews and annotations where somebody else has done the work. Unfortunately a reviewer or annotator often writes his piece from a particular standpoint, rather than providing an entirely balanced view of what has been published before. The use of meta-analyses to summarize the findings from a number of small but similar clinical trials has become very popular, but the results of meta-analyses, rather like reviews, are dependent on the selection of papers or trials made by the author. There is the inevitable problem that papers with negative findings are much less likely to be published and therefore less likely to find their way into reviews or meta-analyses, providing a publication bias in favour of positive results.

Conferences would seem to be a good way of disseminating research, but they are usually regarded as somewhere where one meets friends and perhaps tries to impress others with one's own erudition. Sessions labelled 'personal practice' tend to be very popular with general paediatricians and neonatologists, as they are the verbal equivalent of the review or annotation. Nevertheless, they suffer the same problems in that they depend very much upon who the presenter is and what is his standpoint.

Drug company representatives form a significant influence, particularly on junior doctors and doctors in district hospitals. They certainly endeavour to ply their customers with apparently scientifically based information about their company's products. Inevitably, of course, such information is very biased, selective and much of the research is of poor quality.

Pressure groups, particularly those run by parents of children with particular conditions, may also try to influence the medical profession by mailing to them selections of research papers, usually chosen by a member of the medical profession, to make a particular treatment or method of treatment look more favourable. Peers, and in neonatal care, particularly the trained neonatal nurse, have an influence in the introduction of new techniques which is not to be dismissed. For example the widespread introduction of opiate analgesia into intensive care units in recent years has been largely as the result of nursing pressure rather than of sound research data. That is not to say that infants do not feel pain but the introduction of the widespread use of opiates for even minor procedures has been on the basis of an emotional response rather than good research findings.

Being involved directly in a research project, whether as an individual or as a unit, has a valuable effect in raising awareness about its value. It is interesting to see what happens after a particular technique has been shown to be useful. For example, in the prophylaxis for periventricular haemorrhage, the use of drugs such as ethamsylate and vitamin E, although demonstrated to be of value in reasonably well conducted clinical trials, has remained confined to those centres involved in the original studies. Publication of trial data has not been enough to convince others of its value. With new structures in the Health Service it might be thought that management might be more actively involved in the selection of clinical techniques on the basis of scientific and economic evaluations. To date this has not occurred, at least in my own experience, and managers are content to leave clinical matters to clinicians. Whether this is likely to continue in the future is less certain. A more critical evaluation of many of the more expensive aspects of care has been called for, and examples of costly techniques being limited by management are beginning to appear.

It is possible to illustrate the points already made by examining how, in three particular areas of neonatal care, clinical management has been influenced by research findings.

VITAMIN K PROPHYLAXIS FOR HAEMORRHAGIC DISEASE

Haemorrhagic disease of the newborn was recognized as a separate entity from haemophilia as long ago as the 1890s. Some 30 years later the role of a factor, later identified as vitamin K, was identified and the logical step to prophylaxis with intramuscular injections of vitamin K taken. For many years this was a good example of how research had found the cause of a problem and put it right.

After some years with very little haemorrhagic disease occurring, the wholesale treatment of newborn infants with painful intramuscular injections was considered to be overtreatment, and in many parts of the country was stopped. Initially little change was seen but then cases began to appear. Because of concern about painful injections and the cost of needles and syringes, oral vitamin K was introduced. The pressure for this was more emotional than scientific and evidence for efficacy was lacking.

More recently, a number of cases of haemorrhagic disease in children, who were treated orally, has been reported and there is a move back to treatment with intramuscular vitamin K. However, at a recent national meeting of neonatal paediatricians a show of hands indicated that although rather more than half of all babies in the United Kingdom were likely to be receiving intramuscular vitamin K, many of the rest were being treated orally and many were being treated with no vitamin K at all. Despite abundant evidence of efficacy of a particular treatment and its initial adoption, the scientific evidence has not allowed that treatment to continue.

EARLY MOTHER–INFANT CONTACT

Another example is that of the encouragement of early mother–infant contact. Benefits for this have been claimed for at least 100 years. Pierre Budin wrote in his book '*The Nursling*' that he had encountered marked problems where mother–infant separation had occurred and he had made arrangements for mothers to be involved with the care of their infants from an early stage.

In subsequent years, as neonatal units developed, justifiable fears of infection encouraged physicians to react by excluding parents to a greater or lesser extent from neonatal nurseries. In the 1960s and 1970s such exclusion was interpreted as a demonstration of power and territorial ownership by physicians rather than a genuine concern for the infant, and it was at this time that Klaus and Kenell collected together such work as had been done, in their influential book '*Maternal Infant Bonding*'.

It was indeed an idea whose time had come. The book itself is a readable mixture of anecdote, cross-species and cross-cultural research. The authors undoubtedly had a caring yet crusading attitude to their subject. Soon no nursing or medical conference was complete without a presentation of the importance of 'Bonding'. Techniques for introducing mothers to units and involving them with the care of their young babies were introduced widely and uncritically.

While there is little, if any, evidence that this has caused any harm and it has probably done a great deal of good, it is incorrect to believe that such changes are based on sound scientific evidence. Nevertheless, they have been introduced far more effectively than many techniques where scientific evidence has been stronger.

SURFACTANT THERAPY

A final example is the way in which surfactant therapy has been tested clinically and introduced. Over the past two decades there has been a considerable research effort in this area. More experimental work has been done on surfactant therapy than almost any other neonatal therapy to date. Numerous clinical trials and meta-analyses have been published.

The approach taken by one company in organizing its research does, however, give a clue as to how findings of neonatal clinical research might be rapidly and effectively introduced into daily practice. Wellcome, the company manufacturing Exosurf®, rather than confining its research effort to a few major centres, has used an extremely large number of centres, both large and small, throughout Great Britain and Europe to conduct the largest ever clinical trial in neonatal medicine. The 'OSIRIS' trial, which aims to enrol some four thousand patients, has exposed numerous centres to the techniques and rigours of clinical research, which would have not normally been involved otherwise. The company has provided all the facilities and the surfactant for this trial, but of course such largesse will cease when the trial ceases.

Having been exposed to the effects of this drug and seen the research results, it is highly unlikely that clinicians will do anything but continue to use the treatment in their centre, despite its cost. This will lead to a widespread future use of surfactant, which was less likely to have occurred, had the research been confined to a few major centres.

Could this technique be used to do the same for other research ideas? The National Perinatal Epidemiology Unit and the British Association for Perinatal Medicine have recently begun to form a clinical trials group. The idea for this grew out of the 'OSIRIS' trial. All neonatologists and obstetricians in the United Kingdom have been approached, and to date 50% of them have replied. The majority of these want to take part in future clinical trials in perinatal medicine. By encouraging and fostering such a development, neonatal units large and small up and down the country will learn by their involvement in research, will become convinced of its value, and continue to use scientifically based methods in their daily practice. Research findings will no longer be the property of the few but will be widely owned and used.

General discussion III

Rupert Fawdry (Obstetrician, Milton Keynes)   It is vitally important that research does get publicized. Those who fund units like the National Perinatal Epidemiology Unit and Birthright, should be encouraged to consider the costs of the production of papers and publications. If you are going to spend a lot of money on projects you ought to give a little bit more on making the results known.

Barbara Stocking (Director, King's Fund Centre, London)   That is a very positive suggestion. Much more has to be done to get the information out, to get the whole change process started. This is beginning to be recognized by some of the funding bodies; it was mentioned earlier that the Joseph Rowntree Memorial Trust is now employing its own publicity officer to help researchers rewrite their results in ways that can influence policy. They are also using well-known journalists to interpret research results to get the message targeted to the relevant people. This is a move that is going to be encouraged by the changes in the NHS, with purchasers needing good information. More research results will need to be written in ways that are usable by people who are not expert in the field. Some researchers may be good at it, but others are not and the issue is how we build this into the research process. Perhaps we should institute a marketing post into research units. The funding bodies will have to recognize this and allocate funds for this purpose. However, we must remember that marketing can sell things which are not of any value.

Rona Campbell (National Perinatal Epidemiology Unit, Oxford)   It is vitally important that research is made available in forms that can be used. There are a lot of people doing interesting and useful research who do not have access to a database of similar research.

Wendy Savage (Obstetrician, London)   Marion Hall quoted McKinlay who said that the adoption of an innovation has more to do with the power interests of those sponsoring it than the intrinsic value which is based on empirical research. Caroline Flint's presentation focused on a lot of

153

the emotional barriers which occur when trying to get an innovation going. Ultrasound has been accepted into practice as a routine, and women now think that they are being deprived if they are not offered a technique which is offered to everybody else.

That made me think that the influence of manufacturers of equipment is an important factor in determining how policies and practice are changed. Every week I get an invitation to go to a meeting about transcervical endometrial resection. Although this may be a great advance, the research on which this is based has followed women up for not more than three years, yet every gynaecologist in the UK is being targeted to go on these kind of training courses. What follows will require the buying of equipment that costs a great deal of money, so how are we going to make sure that good research really is able to fight against this kind of commercial interest? How in the 1990s can we actually make sure that decent research does influence policy?

Marion Hall (Obstetrician, Aberdeen) I think this is a very important issue and theoretically the purchaser/provider split might address it, but I have no great confidence that it will, because the way in which the purchasers will get their advice has not been set up properly. Purchasers are businessmen and I think there is a great danger that they will end up making choices about what they will buy on the basis of business principles rather than the ethics of the treatment or the health needs of the population.

Alan Knight who proposed the internally managed market in the purchaser/provider split, did not propose that it should be implemented wholesale but proposed that there should be pilot projects which could be properly evaluated. What constitutes proper evaluation?

In transcervical endometrial resection such evaluation should be by randomized controlled trials of women who would be prepared to have a hysterectomy, to whom the endometrial operation could be offered as an alternative. The problem is that if you offer it openly, what you will get is all sorts of people who would never dream of having a hysterectomy having endometrial ablation. It is then not surprising perhaps that the results look good. In addition you need long-term follow up because of the possible adverse outcomes in terms of pregnancy or endometrial carcinoma following the endometrial resection.

Iain Chalmers (Epidemiologist, Oxford) One of the things that perturbed me when I became an examiner of the Royal College of General Practitioners (RCGP) was finding the inability of GP trainees to understand and read scientific papers. The examiners for the Membership of the RCGP set up a specific paper called 'The Critical Reading Question'.

This has had an immediate and formative effect and shows what you can do with an examination; MRCGP trainees actually have to learn the ability to read papers and study them critically.

I do not think that managers are always concerned only with economics; they are very concerned about patients' benefits but quite often in the past they have been deceived by their professional advisers when they have been told that a particular line of treatment is the right one. There has been a stand-off agreement between managers and doctors in which managers did not interfere with doctors and doctors would not bring clinical problems to managers who they expected to run the household. We are now entering a new era; managers are becoming much more concerned with the business of providing health care. To do that they will be the people who are likely to use the evidence with which they can come to the conclusions they want. I think we must build a base of people who understand much more of the evidence and how to assess it.

Professor Robert Dingwall (Sociologist, Nottingham) It is very important that you preserve your basic research capacity and that things get done because they make good scientific sense even if you don't have an immediate contractual use for them. A specific example is that providers' studies in obstetrics and midwifery have pushed the independent scientific base in research downstream. We must preserve the capacity for undertaking independent scientific work which is not driven by the short-term needs and interests of particular consumers.

Carolyn Roach (Midwife, London) A number of researchers have actually called attention to the factors which either favour or militate against critical enquiry. I speak as a midwife concerned that as a profession, we have reached the point where we are beginning to explore our practice and the way in which our practice impinges on the receivers of the care as well as other professionals. At a time when the funds for research are getting scarce, I would like to ask how we actually create that climate within a hospital setting for midwives (who have not been prime researchers or investigators in the past) to be funded. The interdisciplinary practice of research might actually be reaching a very critical point and I am not optimistic about the purchaser/provider scheme providing help. From the point of view of the purchaser, education and research actually are not very cost-effective, in the short term; this worries me as a woman and as a midwife.

Rosemary Jenkins (Royal College of Midwives) What is there in the application of rational decision-making in the policy-making process that leads to the rejection of good research? Professor Cooke talked about the vitamin K issue which was good research with a good outcome yet he indicated a group that is not using it. The NHS probably does not apply any rationalization to that decision; should we assess if it is valid to look rationally at the cost-effectiveness of that, examining cost–benefits as well and help make a rational decision for that particular issue?

Professor Richard Cooke (Paediatrician, Liverpool) I gave that particular example because it showed that where there was reasonably well conducted research to guide what one should do, there was still a completely random approach to doing it. If you put information in front of people, it is not the quality of the information that tempts them to take it up in their practices, but their own beliefs and their own values at that particular time. I do not know that publicizing research work better is necessarily going to help.

Rosemary Jenkins It is likely that people will make random decisions, but is there not a case for rational decision-making which can still lead to the rejection of the use of good research?

Professor Cooke Probably this is being done on the basis of the fact that you could prevent it but it would be too expensive to do so; that already happens in a covert way in the Health Service. Children who could benefit from intensive care do not get it, and it probably happens with other forms of high technology therapy. The NHS limits the access to care by making it difficult to get; other health systems make it too expensive for most people to get. We say it is free to everybody if you can get it but it is very difficult to get it in some cases. So all health care is rationed by one system or other, inevitably.

People are now saying we want information and we are getting pressure from the managerial side indicating that it is very important that we have research trials done, and data must be aggregated in a way that we can use. Even the Department of Health seems to be moving slightly. There is work on a number of effectiveness policies that will try to summarize evidence over a range of areas. It will also show just how much is unknown about the effectiveness and cost-effectiveness of care. Up to now nobody has been very interested in whether clinical care has been shown to be effective or not. Now purchasers are beginning to ask questions; this means we might get some money to get more of that research done.

Rona MacCandish (Midwife, National Perinatal Epidemiology Unit) What we are learning is that through the 1990s we need to keep up the evaluation of evidence. That which is produced is not going to be for all time; health care is a dynamic institution, socially, professionally, and personally. Information about effectiveness must be a continuum. No matter how convinced professionals are, they must be prepared to be challenged and to move on. I hope that is what the 1990s will do for research in midwifery and obstetrics.

Section 4
The way forward

16
Maternity services after 1992

Rosemary Jenkins

IMPORTANT ISSUES OF 1992

It is particularly appropriate to look intently at 1992 in order to pinpoint the particular changes in that year that will impinge upon the provision of maternity care. There are three issues which must be considered, separate in themselves but which intertwine to create a pressure upon the policy-makers which is likely to influence the way maternity services are organized. These are the NHS reforms, the findings of the 1991 census and the Single European Act.

The NHS reforms

In 1992 we will see the second wave of NHS trusts. It will be possible to look back over a year to see the problems and initial achievements of the trusts that came into being at the beginning of April 1991. We are likely to see the setting up of an even larger tranche of self-governing services, including possibly the first self-governing maternity service in Liverpool. Considerable numbers of maternity unit staff will be faced with working under terms and conditions of service set by their local employer even when this is introduced slowly. They will be working for employers who will be able to make autonomous decisions about the level of care they wish to provide, the standards of that care and the staff grades they wish to employ. The employers will have upon them the two external pressures of needing to retain a competitive edge while remaining financially viable. These are pressures which were much more overt in the private than in the public sector.

This is not necessarily bad; it is the way successful companies operate. The successful company operates in a tight financial framework, has usually secured amicable industrial relations and above all produces a product that its customers want and need. In the words of the British Standards Institute, a product that is 'fit for the purpose and safe in use'[1].

In 1992 there will also be a movement away from block contracts for health care to more explicit contracts which will need to specify agreed quality measures as well as the cost and volume of services required. It will be the second year of patient choice and audit being part of the explicit agenda for health care. District health authorities will be in the second year of determining health care needs and purchasing services to meet those needs within the financial limitation placed upon them by the new funding mechanism. It will be the second year without the protection that Crown immunity once offered to health services, and the third year that the Health Service has been required to offer to medical staff the Crown Indemnity that all other staff have enjoyed, with the responsibility for that devolved upon the providers of health care.

Census information and demographic change

The phrase Black Hole took on quite a different meaning in the late 1980s. Health service managers and civil servants began to use the phrase to describe the acute skills shortage that would hit the NHS by the mid-1990s. That point has not yet been reached and indeed other unforeseen factors have perhaps lessened the anticipated problems. From a general observation by national officers of the Royal College of Midwives, fewer women are leaving work after maternity leave and the workforce seems to be more static although there are still areas of extreme difficulty. There are however other demographic changes which will impinge upon health care provision, and particularly upon the provision of maternity care.

Peter Wormald, Registrar General for England and Wales has predicted some of the Census findings. There will be an increase in unmarried cohabitation, more children born out of wedlock, more one-parent families. Mr Wormald also went on to say that there will be 'change in the age balance with a fall in those under 16 and a rise in the over 80s'[2]. It is also anticipated that 'by the year 2000 there will be one pensioner to each employee in Europe'[3].

The Single European Act

The purpose behind the Treaty of Rome was to create a large area with a common economic policy. The mechanism for producing this is the creation of a single market combined with progressive convergence of the economic policies of the member states. In 1985, the member states committed themselves to completing this work by the end of 1992. In the United Kingdom the statutory framework for this change was introduced with the Single European Act (1987). This Act has four concepts: the free movement of citizens, goods, capital and services.

There is no specific mention of health care in the Act, but the provision to encourage free movement of services is likely to be broad enough to encompass health care if there is a will to do so. It would seem that the lack of specific mention means that member states are not particularly interested in a bringing together of their health care delivery systems. However, in some respects there are already some important European influences upon the maternity services in the form of reciprocal training arrangements, for example the European Community Midwives Directive[4].

EFFECTS ON THE MATERNITY SERVICES

The second part of this chapter will address the potential of these three issues for changing the maternity services in a more powerful way than we have experienced before.

Setting priorities in care

There is not, and never has been, a health care system with sufficient funding to meet the perceived health care need. All systems therefore, unconnected to the decision about how much of gross national product should be devoted to health care, have some rationing system. The NHS has depended upon two outstanding mechanisms: the waiting list, and the lip service that is paid to finding out what people's true health status is. The White Paper 'Working for Patients'[5] effectively called a halt to these. The waiting list is to be reduced and health authorities are now charged with identifying health care need.

The Maternity Services have not been subjected to either of these priority mechanisms. They have always acted as an emergency service and cannot turn away the work presented to them. The NHS cuts of the past few years have left them relatively unscathed but this is unlikely to be the case in the future. To translate this into crude business terms, a company, to be successful, cannot continue to put unquestioned resources into one department while at the same time requiring strict financial controls in others. We are still, quite rightly, going to be expected to offer care to all who need it but will have to be much more selective in how that care is given.

Appropriate care

Health professionals must rethink much of what is on offer in maternity care at present, as well as their own attitudes to that care. Marion Hall's paper has discussed antenatal care. What other care should we be appraising? Midwives are beginning to offer selective rather than routine postnatal visiting. But that is for at least ten days after delivery. In France women receive care for only five days, but it is in expensive-to-run maternity units. The outcomes are very little different. The French seem to be as healthy as we are. When we become a part of a single market, and if that is extended to health care, these inter-country differences will become much more apparent to the managers of the new NHS businesses.

NHS trust directors are likely to need a firm medical and economic appraisal before the introduction of expensive technology. But first and foremost the organization of care must be appropriate to the needs of the women using the service. To quote again the British Standards Institute[1] a quality service is 'the service provided or product designed and constructed to satisfy the customer needs'. If we had been listening to these messages in the past, much more care would now be community-based, care would have been organized to give continuity and women would know the professionals who were delivering their babies[6].

If maternity care is to be consumer-based care, it must be subjected to a fundamental reorganization, affecting the working practices and roles of all the professional groups.

Staffing the services

The long-held view of the Royal College of Midwives is that the health services are failing to use the skills of midwives properly; a view based upon evidence of many years[7,8]. A staffing structure that is designed to match the right skills level to the health care need will become an overwhelming priority for managers with financial targets. The further requirement to rationalize the hours of junior doctors in the hospital service, and the increased pressure that the family practitioner services are facing as the number of elderly increases begin to create the imperative for change. The three professional groups of obstetricians, midwives and GPs will be forced by circumstance, if they do not do it willingly, to find common ground in their discussions about the relative worth and responsibility of each. Duplication of skills cannot remain on the health care agenda much longer.

So far this debate about the roles of midwives and their medical colleagues has been about shifting responsibility from doctors to midwives. Managers are contemplating another shift downwards to the new Health Care Assistant. Whereas medical attention has always been directed towards providing the highest possible level of expertise in any situation, the emphasis seems now to be on providing the least possible level of expertise to give a desired outcome. The imperative upon health professionals to monitor and audit health care outcomes will be clear; the present systems of perinatal and maternal mortality will be too crude to identify the subtle changes that skill mix alterations will bring about.

European influence may bring about further changes in the staffing structure of maternity services. Staffing costs represent the greatest proportion of revenue expenditure, and savings in this area can seem very attractive to a hard-pressed manager. There has been free movement of midwives in the EC since 1981 but this has not resulted in significant movement of personnel; however there has been little incentive to recruit from abroad except to bolster staffing in areas of shortage. Each NHS trust and directly managed unit will now be required to operate in a businesslike way. It may become very attractive to recruit equally skilled midwives from countries where their pay is lower. Based solely upon the barrier of language, this is likely to result in an inflow of English-speaking midwives from elsewhere but will not offer the same opportunities to the British midwife whose second language is likely to be indeterminate school French.

Midwives and obstetricians ignore European pressures on staffing and competition at their peril. Already the Institute of Health Service Management, the European Health Care Management Association and the National Association of Health Authorities and Trusts have held their first joint seminar and are preparing a joint European Handbook[9].

Competition

Talking to midwives around the United Kingdom one finds complacency about the role competition will play in the health services in the future. Where there is only one maternity unit where will the pressures be? Women do want to have their care as locally based as possible. But it has also been shown historically that if a service offers something outstanding they will then travel. Women travelled to central France to receive their care from Michel Odent. If they see an attractive option for care elsewhere those who can, may go.

Competition does not end there. NHS maternity care will be available from whichever agency receives a contract to provide care. A Swedish company is already conducting feasibility studies on the provision of hotel rather than hospital services for some treatments. Postnatal care could lend itself to this. In an attempt to offload the burden of Crown indemnity could not a Trust and DHA combine to offer health care contracts to self-employed obstetricians and midwives who must therefore meet their own indemnity costs? The professions in such circumstances could be in direct competition, dependent for their income on women's choices about the care they want to receive. To succeed in a competitive market, however, the professions are constrained by codes on advertising that do not bind the health service manager or the private health care company.

A source of competition already asserting itself is the general practitioner who has employed a practice midwife and is offering a service, usually for antenatal and postnatal care as an alternative to the service provided by the health authority.

The lesson to be learned from the competitive market is that the organization most likely to succeed is the one that conforms to customer requirements. In the maternity services, the first group, GP practice, NHS trust, directly-managed unit, obstetrician or midwife-led care, that offers continuity of care is likely to become the market leader.

CONCLUSIONS

The future maternity services will be affected by the changes in the NHS which are likely to require an appraisal of the organization and staffing of the services. The pressures in future will be to achieve outcomes of care for least cost. Appropriate care as demonstrated by research and other sound empirical evidence, and as required by service users will be required by the new NHS management, influenced as it will be by the pressures of financial constraint and competition.

Managers will look to staffing by minimum grades to achieve desired outcomes of care, and the opportunities for them to do this will not lie solely with redistribution of work through the professions, but will include the use of staff who have received minimum preparation for their role or staff from the wider European market.

The professional role in audit, particularly in partnership with the consumers of the service will be the most effective way to maintain desired quality.

Competition in the maternity services is probably inevitable. This can take the form of different service provision, such as hotel services, professionals in direct competition with each other or geographical competition for those women able and willing to travel for the care they want.

REFERENCES

1. British Standards Institute. (1988). *BS 5750: A Positive contribution to better business*, p. 4. (London: BSI Quality Assurance)
2. Weaver, M. (1991). Why Mr Wormald wants an answer. *Daily Telegraph.* 19th April. p. 19
3. van Wijk, C. and Wilder, G. (1991). Europe and the Health Service: 1992 and beyond. *Beachcroft Stanley's Health Law Bulletin.* No. 10, pp. 7–8
4. European Community Midwives Directive 80/155/EEC Article 4
5. Department of Health. (1989). White Paper. *Working for Patients.* (London: HMSO)
6. Flint, C. and Poulengeris, K. (1987). *The 'Know Your Midwife' Report.* (London: 49, Peckarmans Wood, SE26 6RZ)
7. Brooks, F., Long, A. and Rathwell, T. (1987). *Midwives Perceptions on the State of Midwifery.* (Leeds: Nuffield Centre for Health Services Studies, University of Leeds)
8. Robinson, S., Golden, J. and Bradley, S. (1983). *A Study of the Role and Responsibilities of the Midwife.* (London: Nursing Education Research Unit, Chelsea College, University of London)
9. May, A. (1991). Language problems on the way to Europe's centre. *The Health Service Journal*, **101**, 11

17
Changing the training programme

Wendy Savage

MIDWIFERY TRAINING

In the UK midwives have always been responsible for assisting at the delivery of the majority of women, but their professional autonomy and status have varied over the centuries. Midwifery is now at a crossroads and what happens in the next 10 years will determine whether they maintain and increase their professional standards and autonomy, or whether midwifery will become a branch of nursing, with midwives acting as assistants to doctors.

Education and training are the key factors in maintaining a strong midwifery profession, and the involvement of midwives and general practitioners in primary maternity care is essential if women are to maintain control of birth as is their right.

Midwives have addressed the problem of how to prepare for the future, and have already instituted changes which will benefit women and educate midwives for the type of practice required of them in the next decade.

There are today two routes to becoming a midwife. Training of 18 months, following a nursing qualification, which itself entails 3 years' training, or 3 years as a direct entrant. After the number of direct entry schools had dwindled to one by the beginning of the 1980s, it now has increased to 11 in England and, for the first time, Scotland will have nine such schools. In addition there are now three University degree courses: Cardiff (for post-registration students), and Oxford Polytechnic and Newcastle University for direct entry midwives.

The content of midwifery training has changed and reflects the needs of the midwife of today. Understanding and knowledge about a woman's need for abortion and contraception, explanation of prenatal screening, basic genetics and counselling skills are now seen as important, whereas 25 years ago these matters were not discussed by midwives or their teachers as part of their everyday work. Over the last 20 years midwives have used educational techniques to reform their training programme from a purely apprentice model to one in which objectives are defined, time is allocated for specific tasks and the expertise used of other professional groups, such as social workers, priests, counsellors and psychologists, in addition to doctors, to widen the experience of their students. In a study done some years ago, midwifery tutors were much more likely to use audiovisual aids, named texts and seminars than were doctors in teaching the important areas of puerperal depression, psychosexual problems and the management of perinatal deaths. In the latter cases, personal involvement of her teachers with the pupil midwife was much more likely than in the case of doctors in training, most of whom had no formal or informal help in dealing with perinatal deaths[1].

The use of research findings in teaching, aided by the Midwives Information and Resource Service, and the involvement of midwives in clinical research, are other advances which have taken place in the last decade. Statutory refresher courses, return to work programmes and in-service training have helped to ensure that midwives keep up-to-date, once trained. As far as the training programme is concerned midwives seem to have prepared themselves for change. Degree courses will enable midwives to plan and execute research, and to increase their status as experts in the care of pregnant women.

The major problem which faces midwives in the educational field is the limited number of home deliveries, that is, 1%, only half of which are planned, Domino deliveries (3%) and GP Unit deliveries (7%) available for teaching midwifery students about primary intrapartum maternity care. An important change would be to start training programmes with community care and normal birth in a low technology setting, so that the young midwife builds on this basic experience, rather than being exposed to hospital obstetrics first.

TRAINING OF GENERAL PRACTITIONER OBSTETRICIANS

The introduction of the statutory GP Vocational Training Scheme, gave GPs the opportunity to plan training, rather than let it evolve as has been the case in most hospital specialties. The insistence on a half-day release for teaching throughout the 3 years, understanding that during the trainee year in general practice the trainee is supernumerary and not an essential part of the service, regular meetings with trainers and appointment of course organizers makes this a real training programme. Obstetrics is not compulsory but most trainees see this as an important area and try to do a 6-month post, sometimes as an extra to the 3-year course.

Anecdotal evidence that trainees are unhappy about the average obstetrics post is widespread, and evidence from studies which have looked at the hours worked and the psychological impact of training in hospital posts[2-4] have documented the stress experienced by young doctors in general. An average working week of 83 hours would not be tolerated in any profession other than a hierarchical one like medicine, nor would a statement of intent to achieve a 72-hour week be seen as a breakthrough[5].

Dr Lindsay Smith has done a questionnaire study of a 25% random sample of GP trainees to see what they think about their training. Table 1 shows some of his results. Does the 6-month training post achieve its (unstated) objective of preparing the GP for taking part in maternity care? These results suggest that it does not, although the majority of trainees see maternity care as a part of general practice with over a third wishing to do intrapartum care[6].

Over half the trainees said that the 6-month post discouraged them from doing maternity care and this bears out my observations as an

Table 1 Assessment of 775 GP trainees (371 male, 382 female, 22 not recorded; data taken from ref. 6)

Does 6-month post encourage you to go into GP maternity care?	Encourage	24.7%
	Discourage	58.5%
How important is obstetric training for GP?	Essential	78.0%
	Inessential	10.4%
Self-assessment of competence		
Palpate pregnant abdomen		80%
Vaginal examination in labour		61%
Artificial rupture of membranes		56%
Spontaneous vertex delivery on own		51%
Interpret cardiotocogram		60%
Perform low forceps		25%
Manage severe postpartum haemorrhage		42%
Resuscitate newborn		50%
Intubate newborn		37%
Site an intravenous drip		60%

examiner for the Diploma of the Royal College of Obstetricians and Gynaecologists. In particular, intrapartum care was seen by those candidates that I examined over the period 1982–5 as dangerous, and the prevailing attitude was one of anxiety. In discussion with obstetricians who were my fellow examiners, they in the main felt that GPs should restrict themselves to shared antenatal care and I gained the strong impression that it was the attitudes of obstetricians which determined whether or not GP trainees felt confident to embark on full maternity care.

In a survey of GPs in Tower Hamlets in 1987, the majority of younger ones had no experience of home birth until they were principals. They experienced conflict inasmuch as they felt they should be able to provide the woman with choice but felt ill-prepared for this task. Luke Zander's initiative in setting up a support group for young GPs has been invaluable.

So what needs to be done in the future to prepare GPs for their role in primary maternity care? Table 2 lists the steps that need to be taken and Luke Zander's thoughtful paper given to the Association of General Practitioners for Maternity Care is responsible for some of these suggestions[7].

Table 2 Changes needed for GP training for the 1990s

(1)	Define objectives
Hospital post	
(2)	Supernumary to service needs in antenatal clinic and gynaecology clinic
(3)	Continuity of antenatal clinic care Attend community antenatal clinic
(4)	Spend some time working as a midwife
Trainee year	
(5)	Spend some time with GP obstetrician to learn about low-tech inpatient care
Examinations	
(6)	DRCOG Joint Diploma
(7)	Log book system

OBSTETRICAL TRAINING

In theory one can qualify as an obstetrician after 6 years training, 2 years plus an elective prior to the membership examination of the RCOG and 3 years after this examination, two of which must be at Senior Registrar level. In practice it takes an average of 13 years between graduation at age 24 and appointment to a consultant post at age 37 years. Another qualification or subspecialty training is needed to compete, so either the Fellowship of the Royal College of Surgeons or an MD is considered necessary.

Although there is a syllabus for the RCOG membership exam and a system for recognition of hospital posts, the training is based on apprenticeship and the idea that by doing a sufficient number of posts in different places, the trainee will gain enough experience to emerge as a properly trained and accredited obstetrician and gynaecologist. In-service training in the form of postgraduate meetings is, in most hospitals, a lunchtime or after hours event interrupted by the ubiquitous bleeps. Midwives and nurses do not seem to recognize the need for doctors to eat, sleep or be taught or be able to distinguish between information that needs to be urgently communicated and that which can wait until the doctor comes round.

A survey done by an RCOG Working Party, looking at the 'Role of Women Doctors in Obstetrics and Gynaecology', documented the dissatisfaction of many trainees with the long hours and disruption of family and social life, expressed by both men and women but did not get the message that the training programme needs to be shorter and more structured[8]. The establishment of a network of district tutors to complement the regional advisers was a golden opportunity to train people for this role, but the implementation was undemocratic and attitudes vary. Table 3 lists some of the ideas put forward by myself[9] and Susan Bewley[10], which we think would improve recruitment, improve training and produce obstetricians and gynaecologists who would be prepared for the changes in society outlined by Ann Oakley.

I believe that midwives, perhaps because they are women, have accepted that women expect a different style of care in the 1990s. The women's movement has accelerated changes for women in society and midwives are influenced by those changes in a way that has hardly touched the profession of obstetrics. The paternalistic style of care has retreated faster from general practice than from obstetrics. If we as a profession are to respond to the needs of women we have to address the way that we train future obstetricians, and stop hiding behind the smokescreen of the fear of litigation. We must address the attitudes within the profession, and I welcome the fact that of the ten obstetricians present for at least part of this meeting we have the president, secretary and a past vice-president of the RCOG – as well as three women obstetricians.

In the USA women trainees in obstetrics and gynaecology comprise a majority in many training programmes, and account for almost 50%

Table 3 Improving recruitment to obstetrics and gynaecology

(1) Shorten the training programme.

(2) Structure the training programme.

(3) Regional schemes to reduce moving during training, and allow doctors to plan lives as well as careers.

(4) Nominated person responsible for regional scheme, full-time and taking part in regular reviews of trainees' progress and adequacy of training and experience.

(5) Consider separation of obstetrics and gynaecology.

(6) Subspecialization spread wider with consultants in ultrasound, medical gynaecology and fertility control.

(7) Hand normal obstetrics over to primary care.

(8) Double the number of consultants to reduce workload.

(9) Trainees should expect a consultant post by age 30.

overall. This has had an effect on the trainers and the training programmes, and I hope that this will also happen in the UK[11]. Part-time training is not the answer, although for a minority of women it may allow training to be completed. We must reduce the time spent in training and the hours worked. I believe this can be done without loss of competence if we look carefully at how to train people rather than seeing them as pairs of hands who will pick up what they need if the training period extends long enough.

CONCLUSION

Maternity care has changed considerably over the last 25 years and one major change is the increased involvement of obstetricians at the expense of midwives and GPs. There is no good evidence that using obstetricians in this way is the best use of their skills, and there is evidence that women prefer primary maternity care by midwives and GPs, a type of care associated with less intervention[12,13].

Midwives have changed their training programme to meet the challenges of the 1990s but both GP and obstetric training programmes need to be modified so that GP obstetricians can undertake more primary care and obstetricians can concentrate on those women who need their particular skills. ·

REFERENCES

1. Savage, W. (1988). The active management of perinatal death. In Kumar, R. and Brockington, I.F. (eds.) *Motherhood and Mental Illness*, Vol. 2., pp. 247–67. (London, Boston, Singapore, Sydney, Toronto, Wellington: Wright)
2. Allen, I. (1988). *Doctors and their Careers*. (London: Policy Studies Institute)
3. Dudley, H.A.F. (1990). Stress in junior doctors. *Br. Med. J.*, 301, 75–6
4. Firth-Cozens, J. (1990). Sources of stress in women junior house officers. *Br. Med. J.*, 301, 89–91
5. Department of Health and Social Security. (1990). *Ministerial group on junior doctors' hours. Monograph: Heads of Agreement*, (London: HMSO)
6. Smith, L. (1991). GP trainees' views of their hospital obstetric training. *Br. Med. J.*, 303, 1447–52
7. Zander, L. (1991). What do we want of our General Practitioner Vocational Training Scheme to prepare General Practitioners for maternity care for the coming decade. Presented at *Meeting of Association of General Practitioners for Maternity Care*, April, in press
8. Studd, J. (1987). *Progr. Obstet. Gynecol.*, 8, 1–15
9. Savage, W. (1990). Women in obstetrics and gynaecology. In Studd, J. (ed.) *Progress in Obstetrics and Gynaecology*, Vol. 2. (Edinburgh, London, Melbourne, New York: Churchill Livingstone)
10. Bewley, S. (1991). The future obstetrician/gynaecologist. *Br. J. Obstet. Gynaecol.*, 98, 237–9
11. Hayashi, T. and McIntyre-Seltman, K. (1987). The role of gender in an obstetrics and gynecology residency programme. *Am. J. Obstet. Gynecol.*, 156, 769–77
12. Cochrane, R. (1991). Women's views of their antenatal care in Tower Hamlets. M.D. Thesis, Cardiff University, submitted
13. van Alten, D., Eskes, M. and Treffers, P.E. (1989). Midwifery in the Netherlands. The Wormeveer study, selection, mode of delivery, perinatal mortality and infant morbidity. *Br. J. Obstet. Gynaecol.*, 96, 656–62

18

Making it happen: the politics of change

Laurie McMahon

At this conference you have considered the 'what' of change; the kind of changes that we would like to see in maternity services and the training of the people who provide them. What I would like to do is to consider the 'how' of change; how to make different things happen. Although the thinking and the analysis about the 'what' is important, without the 'how' you will be merely spinning the policy wheels; producing lots of smoke, but not making much progress.

There are two caveats I would like to make before I begin. The first is that I am an innocent when it comes to the world of maternity services. I have enough experience in health care to know that maternity services are different, but not enough to prevent me from making transgressions of maternity etiquette. So I will ask you now to forgive me when I make my faux pas. My second caveat is more of a warning. I tend to use 'management-speak', a jargon that people like me find useful, but which you may find difficult or even offensive when applied to health care. But you should know that I carry no particular brief for managers in the NHS and am as quick to criticize them as I am politicians, civil servants and professionals, so do not be put off by the language. For once the medium may not be the message.

At the Office for Public Management, we spend a great deal of our time working with real-life managers and professionals, helping them to engineer change. So in many ways these ideas are derived from practice. They are not just folk stories, they are also backed by a strong literature in policy analysis and organization theory, but because the ideas are grounded in the experience of practitioners, do not be surprised if they sound like common sense. In fact, if you think that it is common sense I will take it as a compliment. If my abstractions somehow fit with the way you see the world then we probably have something that is worth working with. What I want to do is to put you back in touch with your common sense, by debunking a great deal of conventional wisdom about management and organizations. We will explore what for you is not a new, but a suppressed, way of thinking about how we can make change happen.

Now that may sound terrifically pragmatic, but I must begin with some theory. That is always a dangerous thing to say because it sounds boring, but when I am talking about theory, I do not mean the tight propositions that scientists prove or disprove. What I mean is all the ideas and beliefs, all the experience and learning, all the prejudice and values that help each of us understand how the world works. It is these theories that we draw upon in thinking about how we should act. It is these theories that inform you about the behaviour that will work best in getting what you want from your professional lives.

The problem is that many in the health service adopt conventional ways of thinking about organizations and management. This leads to changed strategies that simply do not work. We will therefore consider some of this conventional thinking and then explore why it might hinder rather than help. We will then go on to develop an alternative micro-political view of the world, and examine the change strategies that flow from it.

As far as orthodox thinking goes, there are two main elements. One is a view about what organizations are and the other is about the function of management. Let me start with the nature of organizations. We tend to think that organizations are all about achieving a goal, that their very raison d'être is to make some particular thing happen. We then imagine that this prime goal can be broken down into sub-goals and sub-sub-goals and so on rather as in Figure 1. We like showing how all the little things of organizational life, at the bottom of Figure 1, like car-parking policy and fixing squeaking doors, all contribute to achieving the prime goal at the top.

It is a very small step as you can see from Figure 2 to convert these sub-goals into tasks and the little diagonal lines into the lines of accountability. Here you have the beginnings of the hierarchical charts which you all have taped to your walls or, more topically, have stuck in the back of your trust applications. That is the way we tend to think about organizations; as hierarchies of tasks joined with lines of accountability.

The second pillar of conventional thinking is the practice of management. Managers are seen as the people at the top of the organization who have to make it all work. In Figure 3 there is a busy manager on top of her organization. She is establishing the prime goals and the

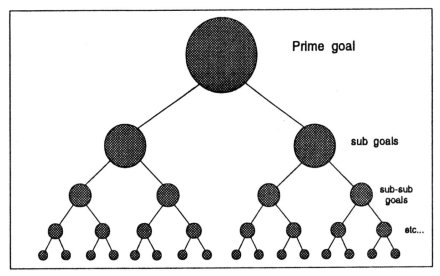

Figure 1 The view of an organization as having a prime goal, which is broken down into sub-goals, sub-sub-goals, and so on

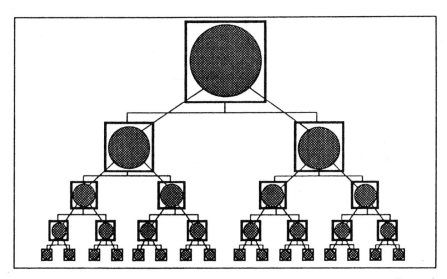

Figure 2 The sub-goals are converted into tasks and the lines become lines of accountability, establishing the familiar hierarchy

sub-goals, she is scanning the environment, interpreting events outside and thinking about what kind of impact they might have within the organization. Then she will use her authority to adapt the content of the boxes and the lines of accountability in order to make sure that all

179

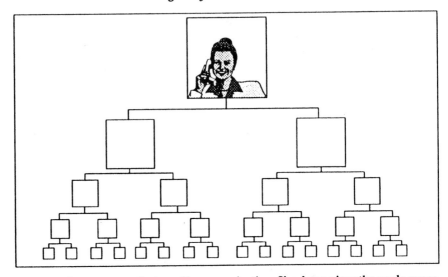

Figure 3 A manager at the top of her organization. She determines the goals, scans the environment, adapts the contents of the boxes and controls the behaviour of those in the boxes

the goals can continue to be achieved. She will also spend time making sure that people do what they are put in their boxes to do.

From these two sets of ideas about hierarchies and management you can draw a very good set of prescriptions about change. Basically, if everything is structured and organized from the top, then it is there that you must begin when you want to change things. If you want to change what is going on down where care is actually delivered then you have to begin by getting those at the top to change their policy or revoke past decisions and then everything else will follow. That is all very neat and may appeal to the tidy mind in all of us but it probably will not work.

Why not? Sometimes the people at the top do not take any notice, sometimes they look the other way. Sometimes they try to invalidate your case, forcing you to use evaluation methodologies through which existing practices would never pass unscathed. Sometimes they seem to delay the decision, asking for more data or a pilot study to be undertaken or maybe seeking the approval of some distant committee, the main function of which you do not understand. There are also times when a decision gets made, but nothing seems to happen, or perhaps the right changes are made, but in an impermanent way, so that as soon as you turn to some other matter then the old patterns begin to re-emerge.

These are ploys that are familiar to you. However, the solution may not be about redoubling your efforts, but about changing the set of assumptions about organizations and management from which you derive your change strategies. I would like to explore now an alternative approach derived from a micro-political view of organizational life. I should make it clear that I am talking about politics with a small p; about interests and power in organizational life rather than the party politics of government. Like all good ideas, micro-politics is deceptively simple. Rather than just tell you about it, perhaps I could take you through a process that will help you put it together for yourselves.

The first thing we need is an issue to focus upon, and although it does not really matter which we use, given the nature of this conference, perhaps we should concentrate on the way that maternity services will be provided in the future. Spend 30 seconds writing down all those institutional and professional groups who you think have an interest in the way that maternity care will turn out in the future.

Even after that short space of time you would probably have a list that includes at least midwives of one persuasion or another, obstetricians, paediatricians and managers. If you have a really good consumer orientation you might have written down 'mothers and their families'. If you have a good sense of politics, you might have written down 'the public', but sometimes that does not occur to professionals who are used to thinking only about their patients and consumers. Perhaps if you are very honest you might have put yourself in there somewhere too. This is the list of partisans.

Next, ask yourself 'How would each of those groups like the services to develop?' Look at each of them and think about what they really want in the future. You will not have to do it for very long before you establish a couple of groups that want the same kind of things and a few that have big differences in their aspirations for the future.

Now go back to your original list and think about the strength of their respective bargaining power. What you have to estimate here is how strong they are in influencing things, perhaps marking them on a 1 to 5 scale. You have now begun to think in a micro-political way. You are beginning to identify those groups with the high scores which have a fairly good chance of getting what they want in the future, and those with the low scores who are very unlikely to be able to influence the way services are provided.

At its most simple, the micro-political perspective shows that if you want to know how things will develop, all you have to do is to rehearse the process you have just been through. Pick the issue, identify those who have an interest in it, analyse the nature of their interests and then consider their respective bargaining power. As Figure 4 suggests, it is rather like a Ouija board in that, if you preclude spiritual intervention, the glass will move according to who has their fingers on the glass, how

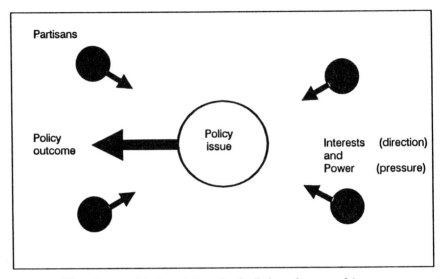

Figure 4 The micro-political model, or the Ouija board approach!

much energy they are putting into it, and the direction in which they are pushing. It is as simple as that.

There are some insights to be drawn from this that are markedly different from those we began with. First, it suggests that there can be interests that exist beyond the boundaries of the organization as well as those who are employed within it. If this is the case then you can expect there to be powerful influences on the nature of maternity services from outside the formal structures of the National Health Service.

It also suggests that there may be quite large variations in the relative power of partisans depending on the issue and probably the place. In other words, you will not get the same partisans for every issue and if you looked at the future for maternity services in Cardiff, they might be determined by a very different set of bargaining forces from those in Camden. So outcomes tend to be issue-specific and location-specific too. You will have noticed also that the nicety of manpower authority has been replaced by a more general notion of bargaining power.

Also there is the idea that much of the negotiating and bargaining around policy issues is not open or declared; it does not all take place at the meeting where the decision is made. Moreover, it suggests that the decision itself is not an endpoint, but rather a middle stage of a process that will involve a lot of bargaining before the decision is made, and about subsequent implementation.

We started with a view that suggested that those who make things happen are the managers and the policy-makers naturally thought of as being at the top of the organization. Now we can see them as being amongst the partisans who are all pushing and shoving around the policy issues. Some of you may remember an album by Dory Previn, called 'Mythical Kings and Iguanas' and to use her words, managers are not on the top where the mythical kings live but down with us where the iguanas play, trying to negotiate to their own advantage.

Critics of the micro-political approach say that it is very difficult to do the analysis properly in a real setting. However, I have always found that managers and professionals find the whole thing surprisingly easy to do. They can use it without really thinking about it, and seem confident about acting on the results without feeling that they have to prove it before they can make a move. It not only helps them explain why things have turned out as they have; why the outcome arrow in Figure 4 is pointing in that particular direction, but much more important, it helps them think how they might begin to engineer change and move the arrow around the dial towards an outcome they prefer.

Once you begin to see things in this light, how to make changes happen seems obvious. Logically, there are only a few classes of tactics that can alter the direction of the outcome arrow. The first is changing the number of partisans by introducing new players on to the map or by removing old ones. Before you dismiss this as impossible to use in health service settings, you should think about the arguments that surround who gets on, or is precluded from, committees and management boards. The second set of tactics is about altering the interests of those involved so that they tend to either cluster around your own position or at least oppose your position less directly. Doing this involves understanding what each of the partisans wants from the future and then entering into a process of negotiation and bargaining. The third set of tactics involves producing shifts in the relative bargaining power of the players involved. To do this we need to understand what makes an individual or a group more or less powerful in influencing outcomes; I would like to explore this.

Understanding the complex interrelationship of factors that determines a group's bargaining power is extremely difficult. I produced Figure 5 years ago when working with a group of newly-appointed District General Managers. We had been talking about bargaining power and after I had identified some key points they talked and I kept adding to it. It is a very messy picture but I am loathe to tidy it up too much because I think that it mirrors the complexity of understanding bargaining power in the real world.

Look over Figure 5, not to explore it in detail, but just to give yourself an idea about some of the things you might have to think about if you

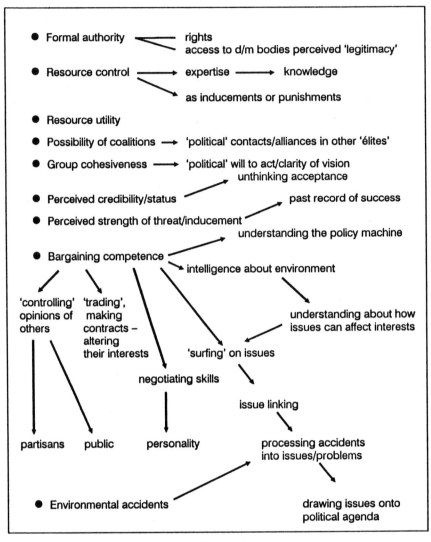

Figure 5 Factors influencing a group's bargaining power

are going to influence the way maternity services are delivered in the future.

My original group was concerned about formal authority, understanding that position in the organization gives access to decision-making bodies and control over resources. Interestingly, amongst the resources they felt most empowering were expertise and knowledge which is perhaps the seat of a great deal of the professional's power. These kinds of resources were seen as levers, as inducements or punishments to influence other people's behaviour, which is right at the core of the bargaining and negotiation process. Note too, that they felt it was not the resources that you have, but how useful they are seen to be by other people that determines their power.

The possibility of coalitions was also important to them, in that being able to make the right kind of contacts produced the possibility of forming alliances with other élites which may not be directly involved with your own policy arena. There is an issue here which may have particular relevance to the professionals and other groups around maternity care. That is the cohesiveness of the group, in that it has to have a clear and shared sense of vision about what it wants and the political will to act to achieve it. Also important to you, the perceived credibility and status of the group was seen as important, in that a past record of success will make a group powerful in a new setting.

Also worth mentioning, is the whole idea about understanding how an issue affects other persons or groups, so that you can see how you can help somebody achieve something that may not be directly related to your own policy setting. The notion of 'surfing', down at the bottom of the Figure, is nice in that it suggests that if something external to the policy setting carries you to where you want to go then you must paddle like mad to get up on the wave and surf on it. If it is not useful then you just sit on your board and bob up and down! Related to these 'environmental accidents' is the whole idea of drawing issues on to the political agenda, and nowhere is this more evident than in the way that professional and political groups use the media.

There is a great deal more contained within this illustration but perhaps a final point to make is that the most powerful force may be the ability to make other people think that their interests are best served by having your interests met. Professionals are very good at this, tending to socialize their public to accept that what is best for the professional group is axiomatically in the best interests of the public.

So, what kind of lessons and prescriptions can we draw from all this in helping you make the sort of changes that you want to see happen in maternity care? Perhaps the most important is to develop some clarity of vision about the kind of patterns that you are looking for and more important to 'hang together' better. Health professionals, particularly those involved around a single care group, are very good at squabbling to the detriment of patients, clients, mothers and the public. You will have to work hard to build alliances around a vision of the future instead of worrying about the differences and the dividing lines between you. Secondly, you have to get to know the policy ground very well. In addition to the good hard quantitative analysis and research about maternity services that I am sure is being undertaken currently, you need to know and undertake the sort of political analysis that I have described here. I think too that you have to learn to be very creative about how you negotiate and trade with others in the policy arena. It may seem unnatural for some of you to negotiate with managers, community groups and other people who are not directly involved in providing maternity services, but that is what you will have to do if you are going to alter the power bargaining map.

All this may feel a little Hobbesian, in that everyone appears to be antagonistic and in conflict with everyone else. But the message I would like to leave with you is one of consensus. You have seen that increasing bargaining power in an organizational setting is more to do with developing a consensus amongst groups of individual players than anything else. This means drawing relatively like-minded people within the system together, as well as drawing on the support of players outside the organizational setting. In the new NHS marketplace, we are expecting customers and the public to be empowered, either directly or through their advocates, the GPs and those who purchase care on their behalf. I would suggest that all of you must make sure that you understand very well what the public and those who use maternity services actually want from you. This may require a reappraisal of many of the professional assumptions, both orthodox and radical, that have been made thus far about what people want from maternity services. It also means that if consumers are to gain power then you have to give up some of yours, which always seems a curiously hard thing for those involved in the provision of health care to do.

General discussion IV

Rupert Fawdry (Obstetrician, Milton Keynes) If a purchaser looks at the cost–benefits of what he will get out of medical staff, he will reject the cost of extra consultants. Although apparently a pessimistic outlook, it is actually optimistic because the cost–benefit of a midwife, who will have an extended role in five years' time, will be incredibly good. Doctors should go back to what they ought to be, the managers, the visionaries, the people who see the whole field and make changes happen, the planners. Morris King said twenty years ago that the role of the doctor in developing countries is quite different from the role of the doctor in the West. We, in the West, are now coming round to seeing the role of the doctor as the head of the directorate.

Jilly Rosser (Institute of Child Health, Bristol) I disagree totally. Doctors as planners can be monumentally disastrous because they have in mind a disease model instead of a health model.

I have a question to Laurie McMahon. I really appreciated your presentation but felt naive listening. I want to get my way by changing people's ideas; and you did not say anything about changing ideas. Lots of midwives think that if we get together all the right research to prove our case and take it to people, we can change their minds and then change will happen. Of all the things you brought up to implement change, changing people's minds did not come in at all.

Laurie McMahon (Office of Public Management, London) I am sorry if I gave that impression. The material I presented about the third face of power, was about getting people to think that their interests are best served by yours. This is the way in which a lot of the trusts and district health authorities are beginning to think about the public. They are beginning to use marketing skills to educate the public about what they should be expecting from the Health Service. A lot of district health authorities do this to stop them getting held to ransom by powerful providers, because they do not want to be supplier-led, they do not want to be led by people who are interested in maximizing revenue at a local

187

level. Most district health authorities are beginning to market the public what they should be expecting from services.

Rosemary Jenkins (Royal College of Midwives) I think both ideas are compatible. There is no point in trying to change anything unless your own case is watertight and you are firmly behind it. It seems that some of the things in Laurie's presentation also reiterated what was said yesterday. I was very interested yesterday about the idea of the iron triangle and the issues about finding where the policy decisions are actually made. We have learned the lesson that we must make our own case, but still have to learn the lesson about where to place it. That is probably the most important lesson to learn.

Sarah Roach (Midwife, Southampton) All midwives have great sympathy for the plight of doctors' needs, for education, nutrition and sleep. I believe that out of this conference we ought to tackle battles that can be won reasonably easily rather than attack the idealistic ones and founder on the rocks of economic necessity. There are some ways we could move forward in education which would be fairly easily achievable with enough goodwill. If midwives' skills are properly utilized, there would be more time for doctors to eat and sleep and to receive education. This would only require some slight changes in attitude, and a sharing of educational initiatives both in the basic education and in the post-basic areas, such as in interpersonal skills and counselling for loss and bereavement. We should be sharing more in quality measures and the implementation and evaluation of quality outcomes. We should examine together what women actually want, the application of research to both our fields of practice which are so closely interlinked, and finally in support mechanisms.

Professor Geoffrey Chamberlain (Obstetrician, London) May I support that very strongly. Those who train together, work together. Much more of the formal training of both obstetricians and midwives could be undertaken in common; it would also shorten the training programmes. We are not doing it in this country because we have different regulatory bodies with different examinations for doctors and midwives.

Luke Zander (General Practitioner, London) I would support the comments made about changing the nature of the DRCOG examination; examinations are an interesting way of influencing the way people think. Most of us who are involved in teaching will be aware that unless something is in the exam, students do not give it appropriate credence. An examination should not be seen just to be testing what people know, but it should be a way of encouraging learning. There are different ways we could do this. For example, much would be gained if midwives were to be on the examining body for the DRCOG, not because the midwives would ask questions which nobody else could pose, but because it would immediately indicate an attitude towards and respect for the profession of midwifery.

The Forum on Maternity and the Newborn, co-sponsor of this conference, has been in existence for 10 years, since the last conference. It has flourished, those who take part finding it a valuable way of exploring new ideas in a multidisciplinary setting. A very noticeable fact has been that with very few notable exceptions, the only group who do not participate are the obstetricians, those who have taken on the care of pregnant women as their life's work. We need to look at the reasons for this. One of the strategies to achieve satisfactory multidisciplinary interaction is to try and ensure it is not threatening to one or other party. In this meeting we understandably and predictably found the session on participation was the only one in the two days where there was evidence of tensions developing between members. Rather than this being a negative feature, I found it a very important reflection on the situation as it exists in real life. If we had gone through that session without any tension, it would have been unrealistic, because we all know that 'out there' the problem is a very great one. What we saw demonstrated in a closed group should not be discussed negatively, but as a reflection of what really happens. We need to explore some of the strategies which have been touched on, so that we can move forward without the antagonism.

Pat Hoddinott (General Practitioner Obstetrician, London) When I went into my GP partnership, I said that I was not going to do any intrapartum care. I now do 30–40 deliveries a year; what changed me were my patients coming to me, asking for home and Domino deliveries. I had no education in general practice obstetrics, and so I started gathering an altogether different set of information from that presented to me as a medical student or as a senior house officer. I started reading books, like Caroline Flint's, and absorbed other information like that from Gavin Young. There is a whole body of information that is not being made available to train doctors in this country. I set about trying to change that and we have set up in Tower Hamlets a support group for young GPs doing intrapartum care. It led on from a group set up by Luke Zander from which many of us got a lot of benefit. Now it has spread to different groups of GPs and it seems to be developing. We can take up educational issues in a workshop oriented way and also involve community midwives. We need to look critically at the postgraduate education organized for GP obstetricians. This is often aimed at passing the DRCOG and focuses largely on topics such as the causes of postpartum haemorrhage rather than being oriented towards the issues that we have been talking about at this conference.

Alan Naftalin (Obstetrician, London) The Hospital Recognition Committee of the RCOG has become important in the training for senior house officers and registrars; it could ensure certain training requirements for senior house officers going into general practice, looking after normal women or low-risk pregnancies.

Wendy Savage (Obstetrician, London) I think that the RCOG Hospital Recognition Committee could make an enormous difference to the training programme, but whilst you have a system which depends upon patronage and upon not upsetting the consultants, you are not going to get great pressure for change from the trainees which might jeopardize their future. As a profession, doctors learn very early to be quiet and not to rock the boat. The students coming in at the beginning of their course are more receptive to research ideas than those at the end of 5 years' training. You put people through the sleep deprivation obstacle course of being a house officer and then they embark on this long training programme. By the time they become a consultant, all but few of them have had the stuffing knocked out of them. I think it is no accident that it is the GP trainees that have taken health authorities to court about their hours; it is no accident that Sam Ethrington who has been running this campaign for junior hospital doctors' hours was a GP trainee. I think that unless we, the obstetric profession, look at what we are doing to our trainees, there are not going to be the kind of changes that women need in our training.

Beverley McCarren (Midwife) I appreciated Laurie McMahon's last remark that if the consumer is to gain power, then the professionals have to lose some power. I was not at your conference 10 years ago, but within the decade I hope that we have lost some power as professionals and given it back to the consumer. The challenge is very much to us, as midwives, to be willing to say 'Well, we do not know best', and 'They are not our babies, it is not our pregnancy, it is not our delivery'. We should take on a more facilitative role so that the consumer can become more empowered. I am glad that we are moving in this direction; we, as professionals and midwives, have had to make this move. I wonder whether one of the challenges to us over the next 10 years might be that we should perhaps be willing to lose some of our own power as professionals, in order to give a better service to mothers and babies.

Leila Lessof (Parkside Health Authority, London)   We have touched several times on the purchaser/provider divide. Providers are undoubtedly threatened at present and feel very insecure; I think there is an enormous opportunity for a dialogue between providers and purchasers of services.

In the inner cities there are many women from minority ethnic groups who have particular needs for services. It is an important thing for providers to remind the purchasers that it is necessary to meet the needs of women with particular cultural, or religious, or other beliefs in terms of service delivery.

Rosemary Jenkins   I want to consider very briefly power and the loss of power. Many people view this transfer of power to the consumer as a threat and a loss to themselves. If we are really going to do that, we are going to have to exercise more skill. We are not going to be required to give anything up but we are going to have to be much more skilled in our work in the future. We are going to be much more needed by consumers in order to enable them to take decisions on their own. We have to reject the idea today that these changes are a threat, they are actually a marvellous opportunity for us. If we go away thinking that, then we can actually begin to start changing.

Laurie McMahon   One of the things that I am often asked to do is to help people manage changes in institutions and organizations. One of the first things you need to do is to destabilize it; if you want to change something, you break the patterns that are already there in order to reform something else. One of the interesting things about what is happening to the NHS now is it has been completely destabilized. If you look at the people in your hospitals, in your district health authority, and examine the names and titles for the jobs now, they are unlike anything that was there a year ago.

The whole system is destabilized and power balances are up for grabs; a lot of power is being shifted around. You must get your act together now, to develop maternity services that you want to see for mothers. This is a golden opportunity and you must not miss it. While it is destabilized, it is ripe for taking if you can get your act together.

Ann Rider (Midwife, London)   A point of deep concern to me is the role of the GPs, the GPs who are not present today. I worry that in inner London where I work, the vast majority of GPs do leave the care to the community midwife. Their only concern is to get the relevant form signed for the obstetric service fee. When I talk to midwives about cuts, this comes up time and time again. It needs to be addressed from the point of view of how can we have continuity of carers doing the same type of caring?

I can understand that the GP perhaps is giving social support to the woman and brings in the medical background, but what does he provide in obstetrical terms different from what the midwife can bring? He is usually a practitioner in normal midwifery; he probably is not even as good as the midwife and his training has not been as good as hers. The midwife relies on the GP for the odd medical prescription for the minor medical disorders. If she needs somebody in labour, she does not need the GP, but the obstetric team. Unless there is a clear understanding between the GP and the community midwife, it is a dangerous situation; I have seen that happen where they have grappled with who is going to do what instead of getting the obstetrician in.

This whole area has not been fully explored; it is one that the Health Committee of the House of Commons needs to take on board for we are talking about duplicating money. There is a wonderful opportunity now to talk about the sharing of normal care, particularly when we have midwives who can take a full amount of that care.

Ruth Ashton (Royal College of Midwives) If we are looking at how to achieve change and trying to rethink education, it seems the principles of training must be: mother-centred and practice-based; that is, practice and education must not be separated but research-based, change-oriented, and evangelical, that is, firing people to move forward.

I believe that looking at the ways in which people are educated is very important but the principles of future education and training must be part and parcel of that process.

Ruth Bennett (Royal College of Midwives) A lot of this discussion has been about different perceptions; we are all trying to serve the same group of people, the women, their babies and families but our perceptions are sometimes different. They could be brought much closer together if we talked together. Luke Zander has already mentioned the Maternity Forum as being one way in which that can happen and the more professionals we can draw into that kind of discussion, the better.

We need to share professional knowledge with women and to ask their opinion humbly about what they want. The word humbly is important. I do not altogether agree with what Laurie McMahon said about power, that if others are to gain power, we have to give up some of ours. We do have to be willing to give it up, but I am not so sure that power is a finite commodity. I think we can actually augment each other's power if we work together. Midwives can lend their power to women just as obstetricians or GPs could. We do have to be willing to share and that is the key issue.

Deborah Kroll (Midwife, London)   The training curricula for midwifes are now changing with student midwives starting out in the community, where they can actually see where the women come from. We have been debating the place of care and the place of birth and I would like to make a plea that this becomes part of senior house officer obstetricians' training. Obstetricians must understand where women are coming from. They have so little insight often into the backgrounds of some of their women. All they see is the woman in the bed in her pyjamas, looking vulnerable; if they went out into the community and spent time with midwives seeing what was really going on out there, perhaps that dialogue between the two professionals would be much easier.

Helen Lewis (National Childbirth Trust)   In the National Childbirth Trust we feel we have done a really good thing because having worked from the bottom upwards for many years and having representatives on local health committees, in the last few months we have finally got together a National Committee so we can work from the top downwards. Now I am told that we should be working from the bottom upwards again. What Laurie McMahon was really saying is that we should be working on all levels.

I very much agree with Laurie McMahon that the NHS has been broken down and it is for us to build it up again as we want with a new structure. Much has changed but one thing has not; we still have all over the country, the Maternity Services Liaison Committees (MSLC), multidisciplinary groups where every interested party involved in maternity care can get together to talk about what is going on and to implement policy at a local level. I invite everybody here today to think about participating in their local MSLC, if they are in a position to do so, and to work at the top at a national level as well.

We have a National Maternity Services Committee in the National Childbirth Trust. I would like to see us invited as a group to work with the professional organizations so that we can work together. There has been a lot of talk about power this morning. What has been going on has been an abuse of power, particularly by the obstetricians.

Wendy Savage   May I share some of my experience in Tower Hamlets? When Peter Huntingford started the Domino scheme in 1977, there were only seven GPs who wished to take part; basically because the others had not been encouraged to do so. We now have a system where we have at least half the GPs doing antenatal care in the community, sharing care with the hospital and looking after their partner's patients. A total of 25% of women are involved in the Domino scheme.

When a GP was using a midwife to do his work, and not communicating with her as a professional should, the Director of Midwifery Services, now the Manager of Midwifery Services, removed the midwife from that practice and the midwives set up midwife-only clinics in the community. So now women have the choice of going to a midwife-only clinic, a GP and midwife team, or a GP who is working without a midwife. Some practices have special antenatal clinic sessions, other practices do it within their ordinary surgeries. We have got professional respect and tolerance in our area. We used sanctions as we needed to if one part of the team was not doing its job properly. We must find a way of solving the problem of GPs and midwives without saying that midwives are going to look after all women because GPs do not have a role. I do not believe that is the case, and I think we have plenty of evidence to show that some GPs do wish to take part in care, are capable of doing it and that there is more than enough work for all of us to do.

Luke Zander How can we achieve the things we are wanting to achieve? All of us were very impressed, not only with Laurie McMahon's presentation, but the charts he presented. What I would like to ask is, how do we actually achieve those particular objectives of process that he was talking about? From his experience as somebody who teaches people how to change the system, it would be very nice for us to know, is this a highly complicated thing to take on board? What does he suggest might be the methods to ensure that we actually learn some of these channels? Is it to employ somebody of his own discipline to come and work in our area? It would be very valuable to have a comment about how easy or difficult it might be for us, as professionals involved in medical education, to do some of the things that you have suggested we should do.

Laurie McMahon If you consider other aspects of your lives you can make little moves, begin to push and shove around a little and things you want happen very easily. As soon as we start thinking about organizations, management and policy, somehow all the native wit that we used to use in other settings seems to desert us. It is really about putting you back in touch with your common sense; the things I said about the golden rules are what I would advocate.

(1)   It is very important to work locally.

(2)   It is very important to work very hard on the values of the mission, to ensure that people from different backgrounds and professions

194

with different views, actually work to determine what it is they really care about and what it is they are trying to achieve. When you do that, with local authorities, DHAs and FHSAs, and actually look at what they want to integrate, it is surprising that what they are trying to do for the people they serve is very similar, given the twenty years of antagonism and rank adversarial behaviour between these organizations.

(3)   Get in touch with all aspects of what you are trying to do because otherwise every issue, every niggle will become a stopper for you.

In summary it is about local work, it is about inter-agency work, it is about inter-professional work and it is also about trying to determine what you really care about and really want to see locally.

You may need some help in starting but it will not be for long, because the tactics are very obvious. Once you start, once you begin to think in that way, you run very quickly.

Conclusions

Geoffrey Chamberlain (President, Section of Obstetrics and Gynaecology)

This has been a joint meeting of the Section of Obstetrics and Gynaecology and the Forum for Maternity and the Newborn of the Royal Society of Medicine. We have heard about the power of obstetricians but that is because of the power of medicine. I sometimes wonder if obstetrics is the same as the rest of medicine; the problem is that obstetricians are trained the same way as colleagues in surgery and medicine on a pattern of disease. Obstetrics however is mostly concerned with healthy women having healthy babies. This is a very difficult area because you have to untwine the entangled lines of the past. I was very much helped by the phrase Ruth Bennett used, 'the augmentation and help we can gain from each other's power'. It has very important implications for the future.

I think every meeting between groups of professionals and women is important, even more important than the decennial ones that Luke and I have run. I think local meetings should go on all the time in one's own place. If they do, we will come together and gradually agree with each other. Those who work together do not argue with each other.

Luke Zander (Forum for Maternity and the Newborn)

The first of these Conferences ten years ago was a very special occasion, bringing together people from a wide range of disciplines, and it led to the establishment of something very innovative – the Forum for Maternity and the Newborn. I was doubtful whether we would be able to recapture that feeling of enthusiasm in this second Conference, but my anxieties have been shown to be unfounded. It has again been an enormous success and for that I thank everybody who has attended. I certainly learnt a great deal and I hope that is a feeling shared by all.

We are at an exciting as well as critical time in the Health Service. Many of the things which have been said give us not only reason for optimism, but provide a challenge for responsible action. There is now the opportunity for many more of us to take an active, constructive part in deciding how the maternity services are going to develop. If this Conference has contributed in any way to that sense of responsibility, it will have been of value for the future.

Index

accountability 21, 54–55, 62
  history of 21, 22
age, average at first childbirth 3
amniocentesis 116
annual report for maternity units 63
antenatal care
  effectiveness of 9
  identification of risk 97, 98
  in the community 193
  research, and content of 121–123
  research, and process of 124
Association for the Improvement of
    Maternity Services (AIMS) 9, 42,
    91, 127, 139
Association of Radical Midwives 127
audit 62–63, 96, 100, 118, 124, 162,
    165, 167

bargaining power 181, 182, 183
birth attendants, regulation of 31
birth interval, UK decrease in 8
Birthright 63, 153
Black Report 46
British Association for Perinatal
    Medicine (BAPM) 80, 108, 152
British Births 1970 Survey 141
British College of Obstetricians and
    Gynaecologists 137
British Paediatric Association (BPA)
    80
British Social Attitudes Survey 6, 7,
    12

Caesarean sections 11, 37, 38, 50, 51,
    63, 103, 119, 140, 141, 142
Cardiff births survey 139
Categories of Babies Requiring Neonatal
    Care 80
census information 162
Central Midwives Board 32
centralization of care 139–141

cerebral palsy 142
  causation of 38, 55
  litigation and 64
change
  and consumer power 118
  and guidelines 117
  and ideas 187
  and incentives 118
  and peer pressure 117
  and practice 117–119
  and standards 117
  bringing about 177–186
  micro-political view of 181–186
  process of 113–116, 118–119
childbirth
  and cultural values 3–13
  medical model of 9
  natural 10
  psychosocial aspects of 9
childcare
  negotiation and resourcing of 8–9
  public funding of 8
clinical trials groups 152
coalitions 185
cohesiveness of groups 185
'commodification' in maternity care
    10–11
community care 5, 170
community health councils 43, 44,
    54, 83, 86, 87, 90, 91, 106, 127
community-based initiatives 9
competition in the health services
    165–166, 167
consensus 186
consumers 101
  and change 118
  future of movement 9–12
  power of 190
  satisfaction of 11
  views of 106–107
continuity of care 18, 127, 128, 129,
    131, 134, 164

continuity of carer 127, 129
contracts, corporate 10, 44, 45, 71, 162
cost-effectiveness of treatment 21
cost–outcome relationships 20, 22–25
Court Report 80
Cranbrook Report 76
crèches, employer-provided 8
Crown indemnity 51, 162, 166
cultural values regarding childbirth
   3–13

day nursery places 8
defensive medicine 64
demographic context of maternity
   care 3–5, 162
Department of Health 51, 52
   and policy-making 41, 42, 43, 44
diet of pregnant women 8
Diploma of the Royal College of
   Obstetricians and
   Gynaecologists (DRCOG) 172,
   188–189, 190
disposable time, women's 5
district health authorities and
   policy-making 43, 47
divorce rate 5
*Domiciliary Midwifery and Maternity
   Bed Needs* 59
'Domino' deliveries 72, 170, 189, 193,
   194
Dutch experience and place of birth
   139, 141–142

economic dimension of maternity
   care policies 19–25
education for parenthood 7
   medical, and research 120
   of maternity services staff 61
   of women regarding maternity
   care 62
EEC directive on pregnant women 18
employer liability 35
endometrial resection, transcervical
   154
Enthoven, Alain 46
episiotomy rate 140
European Health Care Management
   Association 165
evaluation
   of maternity care 13
   of new technology 116–117

expenditure on health and social
   services 9

family
   decline in traditional 5, 13
   lone-parent 5, 13
family life
   changes in 5–9
   participation of fathers in 7
fetal monitoring, electronic 62, 65,
   99, 142
Forum on Maternity and the
   Newborn 189, 192, 197
Foundation for the Study of Infant
   Deaths 9
fund-holding scheme 47

general practitioners (GPs)
   and fund-holding 47
   and isolated units 138, 139, 140
   and shared care 131, 132, 194
   future role of 77–78
   intrapartum care support group
   for 198
   obstetric training of 170–172
   role in obstetric care 9, 75–78
'glasnost' in health care 21
'Good Samaritan' defence 32
GP maternity units 75, 102
Gross Domestic Product and health
   spending 95

haematinic administration, routine
   123
Health and Social Services Select
   Committee 42, 45, 46, 59, 72, 77,
   80, 90, 102, 125, 192
Health Authorities
   and policy-making 43, 44
   as purchasers 46–47
Health Care Assistants 165
Health Education Authority 62
hierarchical format of maternity care
   11
home delivery 59, 60, 61, 87, 98–100,
   137, 139
   and psychosocial factors 143, 170,
   189
hospital delivery 54, 59, 60, 61, 97, 98,
   99, 138–139
Hospital Recognition Committee 190

household tasks, gender distribution
   of 6

incentives for change 118
indemnity
   Crown 51, 162, 166
   Department of Health scheme 38
   NHS 36, 64
induction 9, 55, 140
Infant Life Preservation Act 1897 34
infant welfare 34
infertility, treatment of 11
information
   access of purchasers to 119
   and health care 20–21
   feedback as influence on practice
      117
   Korner system of 20, 28
   imbalance between professionals
      and patients 56
innovations, characteristics of
   114–115
Institute of Health Service
   Management 165
International Safe Motherhood
   Initiative 69
interval between births 8
interventionist ideology in obstetrics
   10
issue networks 43
'iron triangle' 43, 46, 54, 188

'Know Your Midwife' scheme 129,
   131, 132
Korner information system 20, 28

legal aid rules 36, 37
legal influences in obstetrics 11,
   31–39
leisure time, men's and women's 6
liability
   employer's 35
   shared 36
   transfer of 36
litigation, obstetrics-related
   and negligence 35–38
   and recruitment 49, 50
   as proportion of total 36, 37, 49, 50
   causes of 64–65
   increase in 36, 63, 64
   midwives' fear of 51

vulnerability to 11
lone-parent families 5
   and poverty 7
low-technology birth centres 144

Management of Perinatal Deaths 60
marriage, declining popularity of
   32–34
maternal mortality 60, 65, 69, 124, 138
Maternity Alliance, The 8, 42, 91,
   138–139
maternity care
   continuity of 18, 127, 128, 129, 131,
      134, 164
   demographic context of 3–5, 162
   evaluation of 13
   GPs' role in 75–78
   legal influences in 31–39
   paediatric view of 79–81
   policy development in 41–47
   politician's view of 93–95
   pressure groups in 9
   social context of 3–13
   users' views of 83–91
Maternity Care in Action 60, 83
*Maternity Rights: the Experience of
   Women and Employers* 68
Maternity Services Advisory
   Committee 42, 60, 69, 83, 85, 88,
      102
Maternity Services Liaison
   Committees (MSLCs) 83–90, 102
   and NHS review 88–90
   NCT members' experiences of
      85–88, 163, 193
maternity services in the 1990s
   and midwives 68–69
   and safety 60–62
   bringing about change in 177–186
   opportunity for changing 191
   issues affecting 60–65
Medical and Dental Defence Union
   of Scotland 35
*Medical Care of the Newborn in England
   and Wales* 80
Medical Defence Union 35, 49
medical model of childbirth 9
Medical Protection Society 35, 37, 49,
   64, 65
medicolegal considerations 11,
   31–39, 49

Members of Parliament 43, 127
  on Select Committees 93–95
micro-political view of change
  181–186
midwife-only clinics 194
midwifery
  as part of medical education 32
  licensing of 33
  model of care 102
midwifery teams 124, 127–134
  and continuity of care 129
  factors acting against 131
  future for 134
  problems with 133–134
  setting up 129–131
midwives
  community 191
  contribution of 67–72
  facilitative role of 190
  reciprocal training agreements for
    163
  recruitment from abroad of 168
  role in obstetric care 9, 61
  staffing levels 65
  training of 67, 169–170, 193
Midwives Act 1902 32, 34
Midwives Bill 33
Midwives' Information and Resource
  Service 170
monopoly, professional, in delivery
  of babies 32–34
mother–infant contact, early 151

National Association of Health
    Authorities and Trusts 43, 165
National Audit Office Report 53, 88
National Birthday Trust 76
National Childbirth Trust (NCT) 9,
  16, 42, 83, 85–88, 89, 91, 102, 106,
  127, 138, 193
NCT Patients' Charter 88
National Clinical Standards Advisory
  Committee 71
National Collaboration Perinatal
  Project 142
National Perinatal Epidemiology
  Unit 152, 153
natural childbirth 10
negligence litigation 11, 35–38
  and recruitment 49, 50
  causes of 64–65

duration of 36
  increase in 36, 63, 64
  obstetrical, as proportion of total
    36, 37, 49, 50
  neonatal care, future policy for 81
Neonatal Care in Scotland, report on
  80
neonatal intensive care 59, 62, 79, 80,
  81, 104, 107, 147–152
neonatal mortality 59, 64, 93
neonatal resuscitation 101, 103–104
neonatal services 79
neonatal survival rates 79
Next Steps programme 70
NHS and Community Services Act
  1991 81
NHS reorganization 46, 60, 161–162
  effect on MSLCs 88–91
Norwegian Birth Registry 122
Nurses, Midwives and Health
  Visitors Act 1979 32

obstetric history, predictive value of
  122
obstetricians
  and policy-making 59–65
  increased involvement of 174
  interventionist ideology of 10
  recruitment of 173–174
  role in modern care 9, 61, 134
  training 172-174
Office for Public Management 177
Oppé Report 59, 80
opportunity costs 19, 21
Oregon priority listing 23, 25, 55
organizations as hierarchies 178–180
'OSIRIS' trial 152
outcome measurement 22, 23, 63, 188
outcome prediction 122, 124

paediatricians
  role in obstetric care 61
  view of future maternity care
    79–81
parent–child relationships 9
parenthood, education for 7, 9
paternal attendance at birth 6
patient need 20
Peel Report 59, 99
peer pressure 117
'perestroika' in health care 21

perinatal deaths, management of 170
perinatal morbidity 142, 143
perinatal mortality 59, 60, 64,
   65, 76, 79, 93, 94, 100,
   137–144
perinatal mortality meetings 63
Perinatal Mortality Survey 1958 76
phenylketonuria 12, 16
'policy community' 42, 43
policy-making in maternity care
  an obstetrician's view of 59–65
  and GPs 75–78
  and midwives 69–72
  and politicians 93–95
  and research 113–120
  and users 83–91, 106–107
  at national level 41, 42–43
  at local level 41, 43–44
  at point of delivery 41, 45
  development of 41–47
  economic dimension of 19–25
  impact of NHS reforms on 46–47
  influences on 45–46
  national–local links in 41, 44–45
poverty in Britain, increase in 7
pre-eclampsia 124
Pre-eclampsia Toxaemia Society 9
Pregnancy Book, The 62
Pregnancy Care in the 1980s 76
pregnancy outcome 122
prenatal diagnosis 62
pressure groups 9, 46, 107
  role of 17
prioritization in the health service
  19, 54–55, 163–164
  criteria for 20
  need for 19–20
  preliminary attempts at 22–25
private care, and intervention 11
providers 21, 25, 47, 53, 55, 107, 187
  as agents of the community 34
Public Accounts Committee 42, 45,
  46, 53, 88
  Report of 53
purchaser/provider split 46–47, 53,
  54, 55, 71, 89, 106, 154, 155, 191
purchasers 17, 21, 25, 41, 46–47, 53,
  55, 107, 119, 187

quality-adjusted life years (QALYs)
  22, 23, 24, 25

rationing of care 20, 21, 25, 163
redistribution of income 19
research 154
  and antenatal care 120–124
  and GP trainees 154–155
  and midwives 170
  and policy-making 113–120,
   121–122
  and practice 116–117, 119–120
  application of 123–124
  cohort studies in 121
  communication of results of 46, 52,
   149, 153
  cross-sectional studies in 121
  influence of 46
resource management 65
resourcing of maternity services 9
  and allocation 20
  and allocation criteria 25
review meetings 45
*'Role of Women Doctors in Obstetrics
  and Gynaecology'* 173
Rowntree Memorial Trust 153
Royal College of General
  Practitioners 77, 78, 154
Royal College of Midwives 63, 69, 70,
  71, 127, 140, 162, 164
Royal College of Nursing 43, 68
Royal College of Obstetricians and
  Gynaecologists 49, 50, 60, 63, 76,
  77, 78, 80, 172, 173
Royal College of Physicians 80
Royal Society of Medicine 197
'rural midwifery units' 140

safety, and place of birth 60–62,
  97–100, 139–142, 143, 144
screening in pregnancy 12, 16
Select Committees 42, 93, 94, 95, 103
  Health and Social Services 42, 45,
   46, 59, 72, 77, 80, 90, 102, 125, 192
shared care 131, 132
Sheldon Report 80
Short Report 59, 80, 99, 139
sickle cell disease 12, 16
Single European Act 163
social charter 18
social position of mothers 8
special care baby units 80, 81
staffing structures 164, 166

Stillbirth and Neonatal Death Society (SANDS) 9, 17, 105, 106
stillborn babies 105
Strategic Choice Approach 106
surfactant therapy 151–152

Technology Assessment, Office of 117
thalassaemia 16
tort liability in maternity care 31, 35–38, 51
Towards a Healthy Nation 70
training
common, of medical staff and midwives 188
of medical staff 61, 170–174
of midwives 61, 67, 169–170

of new staff 65
trial of method of delivery 63

ultrasound scanning, routine 123
user/provider relationship 16
user satisfaction 12

vision of future 185
vitamin K prophylaxis 150–151, 156

'white swan' approach to research 148
Women's National Commission 68
Working for Patients, White Paper 69, 72, 95, 163